Thyroid Cancer in Clinical Practice

I. Ross McDougall

Thyroid Cancer in Clinical Practice

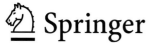 Springer

I. Ross McDougall
Professor of Radiology and Medicine
Division of Nuclear Medicine
Stanford University Hospital and Clinics
Stanford, CA
USA

**WK
270
M137t
2007**

British Library Cataloguing in Publication Data

McDougall, I. Ross
    Thyroid cancer in clinical practice
    1. Thyroid gland—Cancer
    I. Title
    616.9′9444

ISBN-13: 9781846285448

Library of Congress Control Number: 2006940320

ISBN-10: 1-84628-544-5   e-ISBN-10: 1-84628-748-0
ISBN-13: 978-1-84628-544-8   e-ISBN-13: 978-1-84628-748-0

Printed on acid-free paper.

9 8 7 6 5 4 3 2 1

Springer Science+Business Media
springer.com

To the future generation of McDougalls
—Hudson, Logan, and Islay

Preface

The number of patients diagnosed with thyroid cancer is increasing dramatically in the United States, and there are more than 30,000 new cases annually. About 5% of adults have a thyroid nodule that can be felt and between 30% and 50% have one or more nodules that can be identified by ultrasound. *Thyroid Cancer in Clinical Practice* covers all aspects of the diagnosis and treatment of thyroid cancer. The author has spent more than 35 years in Nuclear Medicine and Thyroidology in the clinical care of patients with thyroid nodules and or thyroid cancer. He has published 150 peer-reviewed articles and more than 100 reviews and book chapters, the majority devoted to these topics. The text includes evaluation of a patient with a thyroid nodule. The fundamentals of thyroid pathology are presented. The management of thyroid cancer in adults, children, and pregnant women is covered separately. There is discussion of whole-body scintigraphy with ^{123}I, treatment by surgery and ^{131}I, and the role of thyroglobulin measurements. The importance of long-term follow-up using clinical examination, scintigraphy, ultrasound, and serum thyroglobulin measurements is presented. There are separate chapters devoted to anaplastic cancer, medullary cancer, lymphoma of the thyroid, and metastases to the thyroid. The pocket-sized book provides an easily accessible source of information and advice to help practitioners manage patients and to understand when to refer for consultations. The book supplements existing large texts. Despite its pocket size, the text includes images and up-to-date procedures such as fused positron emission tomography/computed tomography images. There are more than 450 scientific citations from journals. The book should be a convenient reference for practitioners and trainees in endocrinology, nuclear medicine, oncology, surgery, including otolaryngology, radiation, and medical oncology. Medical students, nurse practitioners, and patients with a thyroid nodule or thyroid cancer should find this to be a substantial resource.

I. Ross McDougall

Contents

1. Epidemiology and Etiology of Thyroid Nodules and Thyroid Cancers

Thyroid nodules are very common but thyroid cancers are not. The data that follow relate predominantly to the United States (US). Between 5% to 7% of adults have a clinically detectable nodule in the thyroid and 30% to 50% of adults have one or more nodules in the thyroid when the gland is examined by ultrasound. Therefore, in the adult population, approximately 10^7 and 10^8 have thyroid nodules that are palpable, or ultrasonically visible. In contrast, there are approximately 30,000 new cases of thyroid cancer annually in the US.[1] Physicians should have an algorithm for management of nodules to identify the small proportion that are malignant from the very large proportion that are benign (Chapter 4). Thyroid nodules are more common in women and in regions of low intake of iodine. External radiation increases the incidence. There are families in which there is an increased incidence of clinically palpable nodules and some of these are part of syndromes such as Cowden's syndrome. There are also familial aggregations of medullary thyroid cancer and occasionally papillary cancer.

Epidemiology of Thyroid Cancer

Approximately 1.1% of all cancers arise from the thyroid and 1.7% of cancers in women compared with 0.5% in men are primary thyroid cancers. Thus, thyroid cancer is about three times more common in women. This gender difference is found in almost all countries. One exception to the gender difference occurs in prepubertal children, in whom the incidence in boys and girls is about equivalent. The average age of the patient with differentiated thyroid cancer is 35–40 years. The peak incidence at about 40 years is different from most malignancies that are more prevalent with advancing age. Hispanic men are the exception to the relatively young median age and their highest incidence is more than 70 years and the frequency is 9.2 per 100,000. Other significant differences among ethnic groups are discussed below. Figure 1.1 shows the overall number of cases and deaths in the US from 1970 to 2006. Reasons for the increasing incidence include a true increase that might in part be caused by radioactive fallout from atomic bomb testing and from medical radiation. Alternatively, physicians might be identifying small cancers that would have been overlooked in earlier decades and the almost stable death rate supports this point of view.[2] Small papillary cancer makes up almost all of the increase in cases. The prognosis is good and 6% of patients die from the

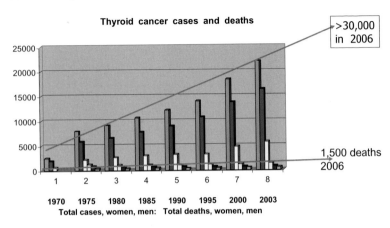

Figure 1.1. The graph shows increases in cases of thyroid cancer between 1976 and 2003 in the US. The increases in mortality are less marked. (Adapted from McDougall IR. Management of Thyroid Cancer and Related Nodular Disease. London: Springer-Verlag; 2006:2.)

cancer but the genders are more equally represented with about 850 women and 650 men expected to die annually (43,000 die of road traffic accidents and 30,000 from gunshots in US annually!). Less than 0.5% of all cancer deaths are from carcinomas of the thyroid. Because the large majority of patients who are diagnosed with thyroid cancer have an excellent prognosis, there are several hundred thousand people in the US who are living with a diagnosis of thyroid cancer.

There are substantial differences in the prevalence of thyroid cancer among ethnic groups. In women, the lowest incidence is 3.3 cancers per 100,000 in African Americans. By comparison, women from Hawaii, Vietnam, and the Philippines represent 9.1, 10.5, and 14.6 cases per 100,000.[3] White and Hispanic women have similar incidences of 6.5 and 6.2 cancers per 100,000. When age is also considered, Filipino women between 55 and 69 years have an incidence of 32.5 cancers per 100,000. Filipino men also have a higher incidence of thyroid cancer with 4.1 per 100,000 compared with 1.4 per 100,000 for African Americans. A multiethnic study in the San Francisco Bay area tried to answer whether there were environmental differences, but no compelling factor was identified.

The 5-year survival for white Americans over time has been 92% (1974–1976), 94% (1980–1982), and 95% (1989–1995); in contrast, the outcomes for African Americans were 88%, 94%, and 89%.

The incidence in the United Kingdom (UK) (1000 new cases annually) is proportionally about one fifth of that of the US based on the respective populations. There are 2.3 thyroid cancers per 100,000 women and 0.9 per 100,000 men. Two hundred fifty (25%) die annually in the UK (25%) and the 5-year survival for women and men is 75% and 64%.[4] The lower incidence and higher mortality in the UK might be attributable to delayed diagnosis.

Summary

Thyroid cancer is not common and there are significant differences in the incidence based on ethnicity. It is not clear whether the increasing incidence is attributable to diagnosis of earlier cases, or a true increase attributable to environmental factors. The use of a staging system such as tumor, node, metastasis (TNM; see Chapter 5) of every new case would allow this point to be resolved. Within one country, the survival is also dependent on ethnicity. The 5-year survival for white Americans was 95% for the period 1989–1995. Over the same time, the outcome for African Americans was lower at 89%.

Etiology of Thyroid Nodules and Cancer

Radiation and genetics are two important causal factors. Radiation causes mutations that can be carcinogenic. There are also familial thyroid cancers that are associated with genetic abnormalities. This is best understood for familial medullary cancer and multiple endocrine neoplasia (MEN 2) syndromes. There is increasing evidence that some cancers of follicular cells are also familial.

Varying doses of radiation to the thyroid have different effects, with intermediate doses (10–1000 rad or 0.1–10 Gy) to tissues being carcinogenic and high doses causing death of cells and hypothyroidism. For many years, the majority of data supported that external radiations, predominantly X-rays, were more likely to induce thyroid cancer. The increased incidence of thyroid cancer in children who were exposed to internal radiation at the time of the Chernobyl incident has altered this concept. Table 1.1 classifies radiation under four main headings, medical, occupational, atomic bomb, and accidental and whether the radiation is external, internal, or a combination.

Terms and Definitions Related to Radiation, Radiation Doses, and Exposure

To define the units of radiation, there are two systems of nomenclature in common usage. This is confusing for patients and also for physicians. The international system (Systeme International d'unites, SI units) is used exclusively in Europe and the non–SI system, or standard system, is used predominantly in the US. There is an increased effort to use SI units universally and in scientific reports. There are also two meanings of radiation dose. One deals with the quantity of radiation absorbed by tissues and its potential damaging effects. The second deals with the dose that is administered to a patient for a specific procedure. Units used to describe absorbed radiation are discussed first. Radiation is energy. The energy of radiation results in ionization of atoms

Table 1.1. Potential situations that could result in exposure of humans to radiation and cause radiation to the thyroid

Major	
Medical	Diagnostic
	Diagnostic X-rays
	CT scan
	Nuclear medicine, thyroid scan
	Therapeutic: external
	Treatment of tinea capitis
	Treatment of acne
	Treatment of hemangioma
	Treatment of Hodgkin's disease
	Treatment of head and neck cancer
	Total-body radiation
	Therapeutic: internal
	Treatment with ^{131}I
	Graves' disease
	Toxic nodular goiter
	Thyroid cancer
Occupational	Medical
	Radiology
	Radiation oncology
	Nuclear medicine
	Nuclear power plant
	Other
Atomic bomb	War
	Hiroshima and Nagasaki
	Testing
	Marshall Islands
	Nevada
Accidental	Three Mile Island
	"Hanford"
	Chernobyl

and that causes damage to cellular materials such as DNA and cell membranes. Energy is usually measured in joules (J) (after James Prescott Joule, an English scientist, 1818–1889). One joule is the energy required to lift 1 kg to a height of 10 cm. In SI units, when 1 J of energy is delivered to 1 kg of tissue, it is defined as 1 gray (1 Gy, in recognition of the radiobiologist Louis H. Gray). One gray is equal to 100 rad (radiation absorbed dose) in the non–SI system. These are quantities of radiation absorbed by tissue. All types of radiation do not cause the same amount of damage to tissues. Photons, including X-rays and gamma (γ) rays and beta particles (electrons, β) are equivalent. Neutrons and alpha (α) particles are considerably more damaging. This is because they have substantial mass. An α particle is a helium nucleus that has mass (2 protons and 2 neutrons) and also electric charge. Alpha particles released inside the body travel very short distances and because of their mass and charge they are very destructive to biologic molecules in their path. An α particle emitted adjacent to a chromosome causes many breaks in DNA. The breaks are in close proximity and are unlikely to be reparable. In contrast, a photon traversing DNA might cause a single break that would be amenable to one of the many repair mechanisms for DNA. Therefore, there are simple mathematical conversions that allow the damaging ability of the radiation to be considered. These are derived by multiplying the absorbed dose by a quality factor that depends on the type of radiation. The quality, or weighting factor, for most radiologic and nuclear medicine sources of radiation is 1, i.e., the quality factor is 1 for X-rays, γ rays, and electrons. The quality factor for neutrons is 10 (range 5–20) and for α particles is 20.

To describe absorbed radiation in man, in SI nomenclature, the sievert (Sv) is the basic unit and in the non–SI system it is the rem (roentgen-equivalent-man). For photons and electrons, the Sv and Gy are equivalent and they are equal to 100 rem and 100 rad, respectively, indicating that rem and rad are also equivalent. In the case of particles with mass such as α particles, 1 Gy is equivalent to 20 Sv, and for neutrons, 1 Gy is equal to 10 Sv. The dose equivalent expressed in Sv or rem is a more accurate index of the biologic effect of radiation.

Next, the units of administered radioactivity are described. That radiation will result in the absorbed radiation to tissues was described previously. In the SI system, the basic unit is the becquerel (Bq, named after Antoine H. Becquerel). It is equal to a source of radioactivity that decays at a rate of 1 disintegration per second. In clinical practice, mega becquerel (MBq, 10^6 Bq) or even giga becquerel (GBq, 10^9 Bq) are used. In the non–SI system, the basic quantity of radioactivity is the curie (Ci, named after Madame Marie Curie). One curie is a source of radioactivity that decays at a rate of 3.7×10^{10} disintegrations per second. Clinically, quantities such as microcurie (μCi, one millionth of a curie) and millicurie (mCi, one thousandth of a curie) are used. One millicurie is equal to 37 MBq and 1 MBq is equivalent to 27 μCi.

Radionuclides of Iodine

^{127}I is nonradioactive natural iodine. The best known radionuclides of iodine are ^{123}I, ^{124}I, ^{125}I, and ^{131}I. ^{131}I is used to treat thyroid cancer and hyperthyroidism and for diagnostic whole-body scintigraphy in patients who have thyroid cancer and have undergone thyroidectomy. ^{123}I is a diagnostic agent used for diagnostic imaging and ^{125}I is widely used in biologic laboratories for radioimmunoassays and for labeling proteins in vitro. ^{124}I is a positron emitter that has value in imaging called positron emission tomography (PET scanning). When ^{131}I is used for whole-body scanning in patients with thyroid cancer, the quantity administered is 37–370 MBq (1–10 mCi) and for therapy 1.1 to >7.4 GBq (30 to >200 mCi). The dose of ^{123}I varies considerably from 7.4 MBq (200 µCi) for a routine thyroid scan to 37–185 MBq (1–5 mCi) for a whole-body scan.

Radiation in Everyday Activities

We are exposed to radiation from common everyday events. In the US, the average total radiation is approximately 3.6 mSv/y (360 mrem/y). This is made up by cosmic radiation, radiation from radon, internal radiation from natural radionuclides mostly ^{40}K, and medical sources including X-rays, computed tomography (CT scanning), and nuclear medicine procedures. In the US, it has been estimated that on average we receive 0.4 mSv/y (40 mrem/y) from diagnostic radiologic sources and 0.15 mSv/y (15 mrem/y) from nuclear medicine tests.

Medical Diagnostic Procedures from External Radiation

An X-ray delivers about 0.05–0.1 mSv (5–10 mrem) radiation. The dose to the thyroid in adults undergoing a helical CT of the cervical spine is 26 mSv (2.6 rem).[5] It has been demonstrated that 0.06–0.1 Sv (6–10 rem) from external radiation can cause an increase in thyroid cancer; therefore, physicians should be concerned when diagnostic radiologic procedures, or repeated diagnostic procedures, reach this dose.[6,7] This is most important in pediatric patients.

Medical Diagnostic Procedures from Internal Radiation

The thyroid receives radiation from diagnostic procedures using radionuclides of iodine and from ^{99m}Tc (pertechnetate). For routine diagnostic thyroid scintigraphy, ^{123}I, a pure γ emitter is preferred. In a normal adult, 200 µCi ^{123}I (7.4 MBq) delivers approximately 2 cGy (2 rad) to a normal-size thyroid; 100 µCi ^{131}I (3.7 MBq) delivers approximately 1 Gy (100 rad) because of its β and γ emissions. A multicenter trial in the US evaluated thyroid nodules and cancers arising in children who had a prior diagnostic procedure with ^{131}I. There were 5 cancers in the 3503 study patients and 1 cancer in 2594 control patients.[8] A study of 34,104 patients who had ^{131}I scans in Sweden showed 67 thyroid cancers when 49.7 were predicted.[9] The thyroids received an average of 1.1 Gy (110 rad). The population included adults and children and when patients younger than 20 years were analyzed there were 3 cancers versus 1.8 expected. The conclusion of these studies is there was no statistically significant increase in thyroid cancer in adults who had a thyroid scan with ^{131}I that delivered on average 0.94 Gy (94 rad).[10]

Medical Therapeutic Procedures Using External Radiation

The doses of external radiation used to treat patients with cancer is usually in the range 40–60 Gy (4000–6000 rad). In the past, physicians prescribed lower doses of radiation to treat nonmalignant conditions. It was recognized that low-dose external radiation increases the incidence of thyroid cancer. The doses used were usually in the range of 1–10 Gy (100–1000 rad).[11] Maxon et al.[12] identified 16 cancers and 15 benign nodules from 1266 irradiated patients in contrast to 1 cancer and 2 benign nodules from the 958 controls. Other studies demonstrated that about 5%–10% of those exposed developed thyroid cancer. Almost all thyroid cancers associated with external radiation are papillary. The latent period between the external radiation treatment and identification of the cancer usually falls within 5–20 years. In one report, cancer was found in only 2 of 700 patients less than 5 years from radiation.[6] Young age is important and the risk decreased in patients 20 years of age or older at the time of exposure to external radiation. Those 5 years or younger are at the highest risk and women are about twice as likely to develop a radiation-related thyroid cancer. The natural history of radiation-related thyroid cancer is the same as in spontaneously occurring cancer. Higher doses of external radiation administered to treat nonthyroidal cancers cause hypothyroidism. There is also an increase in Graves' hyperthyroidism and Graves' orbitopathy after external radiation.[13] Probably the radiation alters thyroid antigens and the immune system produces antibodies some of which are thyroid-stimulating antibodies. Although thyroid cancer rarely follows high-dose external radiation, we found approximately a 20-fold increase in thyroid cancer 10–20 years after the exposure.[13] The high increase is attributable to the rarity of thyroid cancer in normal people.

Very low therapeutic doses of external radiation are also of concern, for example, treatment of tinea capitis (ringworm) of the scalp.[14] The thyroid received approximately 6–10 cGy.[14] Compared were 10,834 exposed children to 10,834 matched nonirradiated children and to 5392 siblings who were also not irradiated.[6,15] There were 44 cancers in the treated group versus an expected 10.7.

Taking all the information related to external radiation, it has been calculated that there is an excess relative risk of 7.7 per Gy (100 rad). The absolute risk is 4–5 cancers per 10,000 (10^4) per year per Gy. From the data available, there is a linear effect from low doses of 0.06 Gy (6 rad) to 5–10 Gy (500–1000 rad). This relationship holds true until the administered dose reaches 25 Gy or higher (2500 rad). At about this dose, the risk levels off but does not reach zero and has been estimated to be 0.4 cancer 10^4 per gray per year.[16] In addition to the radiation dose, the age of the patient at the time of radiation is important. Most cancers arise after a latent period of 5 years and the incidence decreases but does not disappear after 20 years. Women are at greater risk.

Medical Therapeutic Procedures Using Internal Radiation

[131]I has been used for treatment of hyperthyroidism for 60 years. One of the concerns about treating benign conditions with radiation is that there would be an increase in cancers in the organ being irradiated. Ron et al.[17] conducted a large follow-up study of 23,020 patients treated with ^{131}I; 9028 received only radioiodine treatment and the remaining patients were also treated with antithyroid medications (10,439), antithyroid medications and surgery (2661), or surgery (892). The investigators found 29 patients died from thyroid cancer when 10.47 deaths would have been expected [standardized mortality ratio (SMR) 2.77; confidence interval (CI) 1.85–3.98]. The cancers were more likely to be found in patients with nodular glands and to be found within 4 years of ^{131}I treatment. Because of the short latency period and increased number in patients with nodular glands, the small increase in thyroid cancer after ^{131}I treatment of thyrotoxicosis suggests the cancers were already present at the time of ^{131}I treatment.

Medical Occupational Exposure

I am aware of colleagues in nuclear medicine and radiologic specialties who have had thyroid cancer but the denominator is unknown. Cancer mortality in radiologists who worked in the UK between 1897 and 1997 showed no increase in specialists registered after 1954.[18] There was an increase in earlier years but radiation safety precautions were less rigorous at that time. In a different study, cancer mortality was studied in 146,000 radiology technologists.[19] There were 7 deaths from thyroid cancer, 6 in women, and this was the exact number expected in the general population. In summary, the published data show no increase in thyroid cancer deaths in medical personnel who work with radiation.

Occupational Exposure in Nuclear Power Plant Workers

There was an almost threefold increase in thyroid cancer deaths (6 identified versus 2.2 expected) in 14,319 people who had worked at Sellafield nuclear power plant.[20] The numbers are small and could be attributable to chance.

Other Occupational Exposures

The average radiation exposure in the US is 300–360 mrem (3–3.6 mSv). The radiation increases at higher altitude and pilots and cabin crew receive an addition 500–1000 mrem (5–10 mSv) annually. Therefore, a 20-year career could result in exposure to 20 rem (0.2 Sv). A study of 28,000 male pilots identified 5 thyroid cancer deaths, which was more than the 3.6 expected, giving an SMR of 1.48 but the 95% CI ranged from 0.47 to 3.48.[21]

War-Time Exposure to Atomic Bomb

There were two populations, both Japanese, that have been studied. They were citizens of Hiroshima and Nagasaki in whom there was an increase in thyroid cancer. One hundred twelve thyroid cancers (62 from Hiroshima) were identified from 98,610 exposed residents. Prentice et al.[22] conclude "A clear, predominantly linear, increase in thyroid cancer incidence corresponds to increasing levels of γ radiation to the thyroid gland."

Exposure from Atomic Bomb Testing

Testing of atomic bombs in the US was conducted in Nevada. It has been estimated that the US population received 0.5 mGy (0.05 rad) of external radiation from fallout.[23] Since radionuclides of iodine were released, the thyroid was a key organ and it has also been estimated that the thyroid of a child born in 1951 received 30 mGy (3 rad). This resulted in a report from the National Cancer Institute suggesting that this could result in 75,000 additional thyroid cancers.[24] This is one explanation for the increasing incidence of thyroid cancer in the US.

Accidental Exposure to Atomic Bomb

The US tested an atomic device in the region of the Bikini islands near ground level. Two hundred thirty-five occupants of the Marshall Islands were exposed to direct radiation (external) and internal radiation to the thyroid plus exposure to ^{137}Cs, ^{90}Sr, ^{210}Po, and $^{239,240}Pu$. These noniodine radionuclides could cause both external and internal radiation. Ten thyroid cancers were identified as well as 53 thyroid nodules.[25] Six of the 10 cancers occurred in people who were 18 years of age or younger at the time of exposure. There were 39 islanders in this age category, therefore 15.4% developed thyroid cancer. In contrast, less than 2% of older people were identified with thyroid cancer.

Accidental Release of Radioactivity from Power Plants

In the US, the nuclear accident that is remembered best is Three Mile Island that occurred on May 28, 1979. In fact, the maximum radiation exposure to people in the surrounding region was only 0.1 rem (1 mSv) and the average dose was 1 mrem (1 µSv). These are inconsequential. From 1954 to 1957, there were releases of substantial quantities of ^{131}I from Hanford in South Central Washington State into the Snake River, which is a tributary of the Columbia River.[26] Hanford was a production site for manufacturing atomic weapons. Thus, it was not a "power" plant and the releases were not accidental. The general conclusion was that no increased incidence of thyroid cancer was measured. By contrast, the accident at Chernobyl on April 26, 1986 released substantial amounts of radioactivity into the atmosphere and resulted in an increase in thyroid cancer in children. It has been estimated that 1.8×10^{18} Bq of ^{131}I was released plus short-lived radionuclides of iodine. Chernobyl caused a change in the understanding of radiation-induced thyroid cancer:[27] First, internal radiation could be causal; second, although most of the patients who developed thyroid cancer were young when exposed, older persons could also be at risk; and third, the latent period between exposure and cancer could be less than 5 years.[28] The incidence of pediatric thyroid cancer in Belarus, an adjacent territory, increased from 2 per year in 1986 to 6 cases in 1989 to 114 cases in 1992.[29,30] Similarly, the incidence in Ukraine increased from 3 in 1986–1988 to 324 between the years 1990–1998.

Short-lived radionuclides of iodine contributed one-third radiation to those who did not take prophylactic inorganic iodine and for half the thyroid dose in those who took inorganic iodine. The paradoxic higher percentage is attributed to the reduced absorbed radiation from [131]I (half-life 8 days) which was trapped in smaller quantities because of prophylactic inorganic iodine.

Almost all of the cancers were papillary. There is an increased incidence of solid trabecular papillary cancer. Genetic analysis has demonstrated a consistent pattern of mutation. Rearrangements of the *RET* has been identified in 60%–90% of papillary cancers in children exposed to fallout from Chernobyl. This is a considerable increase over the findings in sporadic papillary cancer. The genetics are described later in the chapter.

Prophylaxis for Radioactive Fallout

When radionuclides of iodine are released into the atmosphere, the thyroid can be protected by ingesting an excess of nonradioactive iodine [127]I. The iodine dilutes the radioactive iodine and a smaller proportion of the radioactive nuclide is trapped by the gland. The main requirement is to ingest the [127]I before exposure to the radionuclides of iodine. This is usually not possible. A 130-mg potassium iodide (KI) pill is the most suitable preparation. There are liquid preparations including Lugol's iodine (1 mL, 30 drops, contains 130 mg of iodine) and saturated solution of KI that are effective. The liquid is not so easy to store, it loses potency with time, and is more difficult to dispense. A dose of iodine between 100 and 200 mg reduces thyroidal uptake by 95%. Because of recent concern about terrorists detonating an atomic, or dirty bomb, there has been a run on the sale of KI pills. KI will not be useful for protection against dirty bombs unless radioactive iodine was attached to the explosive device.

Pregnant women are advised to take half of a 130-mg KI pill. The US recommendation for 12- to 18-year-old adolescents is a half pill (65 mg), but because most of these individuals are adult size and they are at more risk because of their youth, I would recommend the full dose.

It has been shown that taking the KI 96 hours before has no protective effect. Similarly, taking the KI 16 hours or more after the radioactive iodine has no beneficial effect. There is a short window of opportunity.

Genetic Mutations as a Cause of Thyroid Cancer

About one third of medullary cancers are familial and there are 3 phenotypic categories. 1) The affected family members have medullary cancer and no associated conditions. 2) Patients with MEN 2A have medullary cancer and about 50% develop pheochromocytoma and 20%–30% hyperparathyroidism. 3) Patients with MEN 2B have medullary cancer and pheochromocytoma in about 50%. They also have ganglioneuromas of the lips, tongue, intestines, abnormal nerves in the eyeball, plus a marphanoid appearance. A genetic cause for MEN 2 syndromes was identified in 1987.[31] Mutations in the *RET* (rearranged during transfection) protooncogene as the cause of medullary cancer were reported in 1993.[32] The *RET* protooncogene is a single transmembrane protein encoded by chromosome 10. The RET protein has a receptor on the extracellular end of the molecule and protein kinase function at the intracellular end. The extracellular segment adjacent to the cell membrane is rich in cysteine molecules. The presence of a ligand results in fusion of 2 *RET* receptor molecules and when a dimer is formed the enzyme tyrosine kinase is activated.

Point mutations in the gene for *RET* are associated with the three syndromes. The majority of mutations are on exons 10 (codons 609, 611, 618, and 620) and 11 (codon 630 and 634). The codon 634 mutation is present in the majority of MEN 2A and familial medullary cancer patients. The mutations are in the region of the chromosome that codes for the cysteine-rich segment of *RET*.[33] A base alteration in one of these codons results in a cysteine molecule being replaced by an alternative amino acid. The cysteine molecules within a strand of *RET* form intramolecular disulfide bonds and the absence of one of the pair allows disulfide bonding between *RET* molecules thus producing dimers. Thus, the protein kinase enzyme is activated without the presence of ligand. This is called constitutive activation. In MEN 2B, the point mutation is usually in exon 16, codon 918 which results in methionine being replaced by threonine. This mutation is in the tyrosine kinase segment and induces phosphorylation of alternative substrates.

The parafollicular cells with *RET* protooncogene mutations first develop C cell hyperplasia and then become frankly cancerous. Curative treatment of patients with one of these mutations requires total thyroidectomy before there is clinically significant cancer. It is of interest that many of the sporadic (non-familial) medullary cancers have similar mutations but they are restricted to the thyroid cancer cells and are not transmissible.

In contrast, the genetic changes in the *RET* protooncogene in papillary cancer are different. The active enzyme protein tyrosine kinase is intact but the extracellular component that binds ligands is lost. That segment is replaced by a fusion gene. These result in oncogenes called *RET-PTC-1*, *RET-PTC-2*, *RET-PTC-3*, etc. The fusion genes contain segments with three-dimensional configurations that produce dimers and when these are formed the tyrosine kinase is activated without the presence of ligand. These mutations are only found in the thyroid and have been identified in cancerous and benign nodules. These are not hereditary. Sixty to ninety percent of the papillary thyroid cancers in children who were exposed to radiation from Chernobyl have *RET-PTC* oncogenes. *RET-PTC-1* is frequently associated with "regular" papillary cancer. *RET-PTC-3* is strongly associated with solid trabecular papillary cancer found in children exposed to radiation from Chernobyl.

p53 is an important tumor suppressor gene. Mutations and deletions of this gene have been found in differentiated and anaplastic thyroid cancer. There is increasing evidence that this mutation in addition to other initiators could be the genetic defect that alters the phenotypes of thyroid cancers from slow-growing differentiated cancer to the rapidly aggressive and invasive behavior of anaplastic cancer. Recent reports identified point mutations in the *BRAF* gene in 38% of papillary cancers and 83% of anaplastic lesions.[34]

Familial Nonmedullary Thyroid Cancer

There is increasing evidence that there are familial clusters of differentiated thyroid cancer.[35,36] This was first reported in 1951 and a few case reports were published over the next 4 decades. It is possible that a genetic defect might make family members more susceptible to radiation. One investigation compared the probability of a second member of a family having thyroid cancer with the risk in families with no evidence of an index case.[37] There was a 10.6-fold increased risk of a second person having thyroid cancer in the former population. A somewhat similar study in Norway found a fivefold increased likelihood of cancer (men 5.2, women 4.9) compared with expected.[38] There are reports of several families with three or more first-degree relatives with papillary cancer and the chance of five family members with papillary cancer has been estimated at 1 in 2 billion.[39]

There is a definite coexistence of differentiated thyroid cancer with heredi-tary syndromes including familial adenomatous polyposis and the associated Gardner's syndrome and Cowden's syndrome. One group of investigators who have conducted extensive research in the field state, "familial nonmedullary thyroid cancer is an emerging clinical phenotype that is genetically heterogeneous, and none of the currently identified genes accounts for the majority of families."[40]

Multifocal lesions and recurrences are more common.[41] Current data suggest that about 5% of papillary cancers are familial. This is similar to my experience with 34 families out of more than 1000 patients (3.4%).

Chemicals as a Cause of Thyroid Cancer

In humans, there is little evidence that chemicals can cause cancer of the thyroid. Goitrogens in doses sufficient to increase thyroid-stimulating hormone can augment the carcinogenic effects of radiation. A metaanalysis concluded there was a reduced risk of thyroid cancer in people who smoked.[42]

The Role of Iodine in the Etiology of Thyroid Cancer

Follicular cancer is more common in regions deficient in iodine and papillary cancer is less common. Laboratory animals fed a chronically iodine-deficient diet develop benign follicular tumors and with time follicular cancers.[43] Most studies show that follicular cancer is more common in areas of chronic low iodine intake. In the majority of reports, the ratio of papillary cancers increases in parallel with increasing dietary iodine. Lymphocytic thyroiditis is also more common in iodine-replete regions. Low iodine potentiates the effect of known thyroid carcinogens.

Estrogen and Thyroid Cancer

All reports of differentiated thyroid cancer with meaningful numbers of patients indicate that women are about 3 times more likely to be affected. However, there are few data regarding female sex hormones as a cause of thyroid cancer.

Geographic Factors

There are data from Sicily indicating an increased risk in regions near volcanoes. This could be attributable to higher levels of radiation. It could explain the higher risk in the Philippines and Hawaii, which are volcanic islands.

Summary and Key Facts

Most thyroid cancers are sporadic and no single cause can be identified. A proportion of thyroid cancers are associated with radiation as an etiologic factor and a proportion have a genetic link. The radiation is usually external and there is a linear relationship from about 0.05–0.1 Gy (50–100 mGy or 5–10 rad) to 5–10 Gy (500–1000 rad). There is an excess risk ×7.7 per Gy. Children exposed to internal radiation resulting from the accident at Chernobyl also have a definite increase in the incidence of thyroid cancer. Genetic defects in the *RET* protooncogene are the cause of 25%–30% of medullary cancers and 100% of the MEN 2A and 2B syndromes.

References

1. Jemal A, Siegel R, Ward E, et al. Cancer statistics, 2006. CA Cancer J Clin 2006; 56(2):106–130.
2. Davies L, Welch HG. Increasing incidence of thyroid cancer in the United States, 1973–2002. JAMA 2006;295(18):2164–2167.
3. Miller B, Kolonel LN, Bernstein L, et al. Racial/ethnic patterns of cancer in the United States 1988–1992. Bethesda, MD: National Institutes of Health, National Cancer Institute; 1996. Publication 96–4104.
4. Kendall-Taylor P. Managing differentiated thyroid cancer. BMJ 2002;324(7344): 988–989.
5. Rybicki F, Nawfel RD, Judy PF, et al. Skin and thyroid dosimetry in cervical spine screening: two methods for evaluation and a comparison between a helical CT and radiographic trauma series. AJR Am J Roentgenol 2002;179(4):933–937.
6. Ron E, Lubin JH, Shore RE, et al. Thyroid cancer after exposure to external radiation: a pooled analysis of seven studies. Radiat Res 1995;141(3):259–277.
7. Ron E, Saftlas AF. Head and neck radiation carcinogenesis: epidemiologic evidence. Otolaryngol Head Neck Surg 1996;115(5):403–408.
8. Hamilton P, Chiacchiernini RP, Kacmarek RG. A follow-up study of persons who had iodine-131 and other diagnostic procedures during childhood and adolescence. Rockville, MD: Health and Human Services, Food and Drug Administration; 1989. Publication 8208276.
9. Holm LE, Wiklund KE, Lundell GE, et al. Thyroid cancer after diagnostic doses of iodine-131: a retrospective cohort study. J Natl Cancer Inst 1988;80(14):1132–1138.
10. Dickman PW, Holm LE, Lundell G, Boice JD Jr, Hall P. Thyroid cancer risk after thyroid examination with 131I: a population-based cohort study in Sweden. Int J Cancer 2003;106(4):580–587.
11. Michel LA, Donckier JE. Thyroid cancer 15 years after Chernobyl. Lancet 2002; 359(9321):1947.
12. Maxon HR, Saenger EL, Thomas SR, et al. Clinically important radiation-associated thyroid disease. A controlled study. JAMA 1980;244(16):1802–1805.

13. Hancock SL, Cox RS, McDougall IR. Thyroid diseases after treatment of Hodgkin's disease. N Engl J Med 1991;325(9):599–605.
14. Modan B, Ron E, Werner A. Thyroid cancer following scalp irradiation. Radiology 1977;123:741–744.
15. Ron E. Cancer risks from medical radiation. Health Phys 2003;85(1):47–59.
16. Inskip PD. Thyroid cancer after radiotherapy for childhood cancer. Med Pediatr Oncol 2001;36(5):568–573.
17. Ron E, Doody MM, Becker DV, et al. Cancer mortality following treatment for adult hyperthyroidism. Cooperative Thyrotoxicosis Therapy Follow-up Study Group. JAMA 1998;280(4):347–355.
18. Berrington A, Darby SC, Weiss HA, Doll R. 100 years of observation on British radiologists: mortality from cancer and other causes 1897–1997. Br J Radiol 2001;74(882):507–519.
19. Mohan AK, Hauptmann M, Freedman DM, et al. Cancer and other causes of mortality among radiologic technologists in the United States. Int J Cancer 2003;103(2):259–267.
20. Omar RZ, Barber JA, Smith PG. Cancer mortality and morbidity among plutonium workers at the Sellafield plant of British Nuclear Fuels. Br J Cancer 1999; 79(7–8):1288–1301.
21. Blettner M, Zeeb H, Auvinen A, et al. Mortality from cancer and other causes among male airline cockpit crew in Europe. Int J Cancer 2003;106(6):946–952.
22. Prentice RL, Kato H, Yoshimoto K, Mason M. Radiation exposure and thyroid cancer incidence among Hiroshima and Nagasaki residents. Natl Cancer Inst Monogr 1982;62:207–212.
23. Bouville A, Simon SL, Miller CW, Beck HL, Anspaugh LR, Bennett BG. Estimates of doses from global fallout. Health Phys 2002;82(5):690–705.
24. Roff SR. The glass bead game: nuclear tourism at the Australian weapon test sites. Med Confl Surviv 1998;14(4):290–302.
25. Conard RA, Dobyns BM, Sutow WW. Thyroid neoplasia as late effect of exposure to radioactive iodine in fallout. Jama 1970;214:316–324.
26. Reynolds T. Final report of Hanford Thyroid Disease Study released. J Natl Cancer Inst 2002;94(14):1046–1048.
27. Goldman M. The Russian radiation legacy: its integrated impact and lessons. Environ Health Perspect 1997;105(suppl 6):1385–1391.
28. Rabes HM. Gene rearrangements in radiation-induced thyroid carcinogenesis. Med Pediatr Oncol 2001;36(5):574–582.
29. Kazakov VS, Demidchik EP, Astakhova LN. Thyroid cancer after Chernobyl. Nature 1992;359(6390):21.
30. Baverstock K, Williams D. Chernobyl: an overlooked aspect? Science 2003; 299(5603):44.
31. Mathew CG, Smith BA, Thorpe K, et al. Deletion of genes on chromosome 1 in endocrine neoplasia. Nature 1987;328(6130):524–526.
32. Donis-Keller H, Dou S, Chi D, et al. Mutations in the RET proto-oncogene are associated with MEN 2A and FMTC. Hum Mol Genet 1993;2(7):851–856.

33. Eng C. RET proto-oncogene in the development of human cancer. J Clin Oncol 1999;17(1):380–393.

34. Nikiforova MN, Kimura ET, Gandhi M, et al. BRAF mutations in thyroid tumors are restricted to papillary carcinomas and anaplastic or poorly differentiated carcinomas arising from papillary carcinomas. J Clin Endocrinol Metab 2003;88(11): 5399–5404.

35. Takami H, Ozaki O, Ito K. Familial nonmedullary thyroid cancer: an emerging entity that warrants aggressive treatment. Arch Surg 1996;131(6):676.

36. Grossman RF, Tu SH, Duh QY, Siperstein AE, Novosolov F, Clark OH. Familial nonmedullary thyroid cancer. An emerging entity that warrants aggressive treatment. Arch Surg 1995;130(8):892–897; discussion 898–899.

37. Pal T, Vogl FD, Chappuis PO, et al. Increased risk for nonmedullary thyroid cancer in the first degree relatives of prevalent cases of nonmedullary thyroid cancer: a hospital-based study. J Clin Endocrinol Metab 2001;86(11):5307–5312.

38. Frich L, Glattre E, Akslen LA. Familial occurrence of nonmedullary thyroid cancer: a population-based study of 5673 first-degree relatives of thyroid cancer patients from Norway. Cancer Epidemiol Biomarkers Prev 2001;10(2):113–117.

39. Malchoff CD, Malchoff DM. Familial nonmedullary thyroid carcinoma. Semin Surg Oncol 1999;16(1):16–18.

40. Bevan S, Pal T, Greenberg CR, et al. A comprehensive analysis of MNG1, TCO1, fPTC, PTEN, TSHR, and TRKA in familial nonmedullary thyroid cancer: confirmation of linkage to TCO1. J Clin Endocrinol Metab 2001;86(8):3701–3704.

41. Uchino S, Noguchi S, Kawamoto H, Yamashita H, Watanabe S, Shuto S. Familial nonmedullary thyroid carcinoma characterized by multifocality and a high recurrence rate in a large study population. World J Surg 2002;26(8):897–902.

42. Mack WJ, Preston-Martin S, Dal Maso L, et al. A pooled analysis of case-control studies of thyroid cancer: cigarette smoking and consumption of alcohol, coffee, and tea. Cancer Causes Control 2003;14(8):773–785.

43. Ward JM, Ohshima M. The role of iodine in carcinogenesis. Adv Exp Med Biol 1986;206:529–542.

2. Thyroid Anatomy and Physiology

Gross Anatomy

The thyroid weighs between 10–20 g (volume of 10–20 mL) and each lobe is approximately 5 cm long, 2.5 cm broad, and 1.5 cm deep (volume of one lobe is obtained from $4/3\,\pi\,r^3 = 10$ mL and the entire gland $2 \times 10 = 20$ mL). The left and right lobes of the thyroid lie on each side of the trachea and they are joined by the isthmus lying anterior to the second to fourth tracheal cartilages. To examine the thyroid, the physician should sit opposite the patient and inspect the neck looking for enlargement of and nodules in the thyroid. I like to palpate the gland standing behind a seated patient, using the first, second, and third fingers of both hands. Alternatively, the gland can be examined with the thumbs while sitting in front of the patient. The size, consistency, and fixation of a nodule are documented. The movement of the gland during swallowing helps define its borders, size, and the presence of a nodule. The location of cervical lymph nodes should be examined routinely. Auscultation can identify a bruit in Graves' hyperthyroidism. An enlarged thyroid is called a goiter and is common in countries where the intake of iodine is low. As the thyroid enlarges, the inferior margin of the gland can move into the thoracic inlet. Reduced pressure in the thorax caused by inspiration, along with gravity, causes further migration that results in a sub- or retrosternal goiter.

Embryology

The thyroid originates at the base of the tongue (foramen cecum) and migrates to the normal cervical position. The midline thyroid that produces functioning thyroid fuses with tissues derived from the fourth and fifth branchial clefts. These bring neuroendocrine cells from the ultimobranchial body that form parafollicular cells (also called C cells). C cells produce and secrete calcitonin. The route between the foramen cecum to the cervical position is the thyroglossal tract. Benign cysts can form along the thyroglossal tract and are common in children. The differential diagnosis is ectopic thyroid caused by failure of migration of the thyroid. Ultrasound can differentiate a thyroglossal cyst from solid ectopic thyroid and in addition define whether the normal thyroid is present or absent. It is important to ensure that the ectopic tissue is not a metastasis by pathologic examination of the tissues for histologic evidence of malignancy. Rarely, cancer arises in sites of ectopic thyroid including lingual thyroid. Thyroid cancer is rare in thyroglossal cysts in children and only 17 cases have been reported in patients younger than 17 years.[1]

Blood Supply of the Thyroid

The thyroid has a rich blood supply. The upper pole is supplied by the superior thyroid artery, the first branch of the external carotid artery. The posterior aspect of the gland is supplied by the inferior thyroid artery, a branch of the thyrocervical trunk, from the first part of the subclavian artery. The thyroidea ima artery arises from either the aorta or the innominate artery. During thyroidectomy, careful attention to the tributaries of these vessels is important, or a postoperative hematoma can occur.

Lymphatic Supply of the Thyroid

A rich lymphatic network drains to cervical nodes that follow the vasculature. Those draining the upper part of the gland follow the superior thyroid artery and feed into deep cervical nodes. Lymph channels from the middle of the lateral lobes terminate in internal jugular, recurrent laryngeal, paratracheal, and paraesophageal nodes. Inferiorly, there is drainage to pretracheal and paratracheal nodes as well as inferolateral drainage to supraclavicular nodes. These are predominantly levels II, III, IV, and VI. There is a delphian node (named after the Oracle of Delphi) in the midline just above the isthmus. Lymphatic metastases are common. Distant metastases occur by invasion into veins within the thyroid.

Surgical Anatomy

The recurrent laryngeal nerves are branches of the vagus and are at risk during thyroidectomy. They supply motor nerves of speech and sensation to the glottic larynx. They have a variable relationship to the inferior thyroid artery and a surgeon should have experience in the variations. Damage to a nerve causes a deep pitch of and difficulty to project the voice. Hyperventilation while speaking results in dizziness. Damage to both nerves resulting in stridor is a medical emergency. The superior laryngeal nerve arising from the vagus is sensory, supplying the supraglottic larynx. The external branch is the motor nerve to the cricothyroid muscle. Damage to the external laryngeal artery produces dysphonia. There are two superior and two inferior parathyroid glands. The inferior glands migrate further and have more chance of being in ectopic sites. Parathyroids adjacent to the thyroid are most at risk of being removed during thyroidectomy and loss of all four causes acute hypocalcemia, tetany, and seizures. Temporary hypocalcemia is common after total thyroidectomy. When all parathyroids are removed (usually inadvertently), one can be autotransplanted. Horner's syndrome from damage to the cervical sympathetic nerve and weakness of the shoulder from damage to the spinal accessory nerve are rare.

Microscopic Structure of the Thyroid

Seventy percent of the thyroid consists of follicular cells and <1% is made up of parafollicular cells (C cells) that secrete calcitonin. C cells are most common at the junction of the upper one third and lower two third of the lateral lobes. Cancers of the C cells are called medullary cancers. The thyroid is largely made up of follicles that are functional, as well as, structural units. A single layer of thyroid cells surrounds a gelatinous core containing colloid. Thyroid cells (follicular cells) are cuboidal and the base of the cell abuts on capillaries and lymphatics and the apex is adjacent to the colloid. The receptor for thyrotropin (TSH) is a 7 transmembrane protein in the basal and lateral aspects of the cell. The sodium iodide symporter (NIS) is also located in the laterobasal cell membrane (13 transmembrane protein) and transports iodide from the serum into the follicular cell. Colloid contains thyroglobulin (Tg), a 660,000 dalton glycoprotein synthesized in and secreted by the follicular cell. It is the site of formation and storage of thyroid hormones (Figure 2.1).

The recommended intake of iodine ^{127}I for an adult is 150 μg/day and during pregnancy 200 μg/day. Fresh seafood, kelp, and vegetables grown in iodine-rich soil are sources of iodine. Iodized salt is a major source. In the United States, the intake is approximately 300–500 μg per person per day. Vitamin and mineral pills usually contain about 150 μg/pill. Medical sources are radiographic contrast and iodine-containing medications such as amiodarone. Populations with low intake of iodine have a range of serious problems grouped together as iodine-deficiency disorders. Seven hundred forty million people have goiter, 50 million children have mental retardation, or iodine-deficiency brain damage, and 11 million have frank congenital hypothyroidism.[2,3] Papillary cancer is more common in areas where there is an abundance of dietary iodine and the proportion of follicular cancers increases as the intake of iodine decreases.

Iodine is rapidly absorbed in the upper gastrointestinal tract and the kidney and thyroid compete for the element. Figure 2.2 shows a whole-body scan 1 hour after ingestion of ^{123}I in a patient with functioning metastases.

The Sodium Iodide Symporter

Two atoms of sodium are transported along with one atom of iodide by the NIS.[4] Radionuclides of iodine such as ^{123}I, ^{131}I, and ^{124}I are used for testing and treatment of thyroid disorders. Their uptake is increased by TSH. Salivary glands, stomach, and occasionally the breasts in women trap iodine (radioiodine should not be administered to patients who are lactating or nursing), placenta (radioiodine should not be prescribed to pregnant patients), and the thymus. NIS also transports thiocyanate (SCN^-), perchlorate ($ClO3^-$) bromine and astatine, and technetium pertechnetate. Iodine is then combined with tyrosine by the enzyme thyroid peroxidase (TPO). Tyrosine molecules situated at appropriate positions on the Tg molecules are iodinated producing

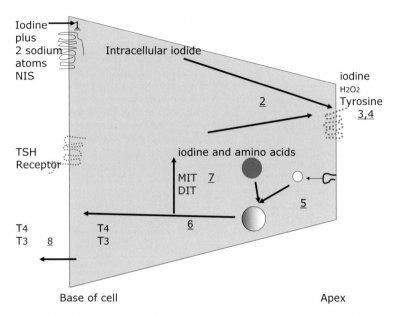

Figure 2.1. Schematic of a follicular cell showing the steps of trapping of iodine and formation of thyroid hormone and the release of thyroid hormone into the circulation.

1. Trapping of iodine by NIS
2. Iodine oxidized to iodide
3. Organification of iodine to produce MIT and DIT
4. Coupling of MIT and DIT
5. Pinocytosis of colloid containing Tg
6. Proteolysis of Tg releasing T_3 and T_4
7. Deiodination of MIT and DIT
8. Carriage of thyroid hormones in the blood

(Adapted from McDougall IR. Management of Thyroid Cancer and Related Nodular Disease. London: Springer-Verlag; 2006:33.)

monoiodotyrosine (MIT) and diiodotyrosine (DIT). H_2O_2 is necessary for organification of iodine. Two molecules of DIT couple to produce T_4 (3,5, 3′5′ tetraiodothyronine) and one molecule of DIT and one of MIT produce T_3 (3,5,3′ triiodothyronine).

Thyroid hormones and iodine are stored in Tg. TSH increases the uptake of colloid containing Tg back into the follicular cell. This occurs by endocytosis. Endocytes fuse with intracellular lysosomes that contain proteolytic and deiodinase enzymes (also called dehalogenase). The colloid containing mostly Tg is digested by proteolytic enzymes and T_4 and T_3 are released into the circulation. MIT and DIT are also released in the follicular cell and their iodine atoms are enzymatically removed by deiodinase. That iodine can be used again

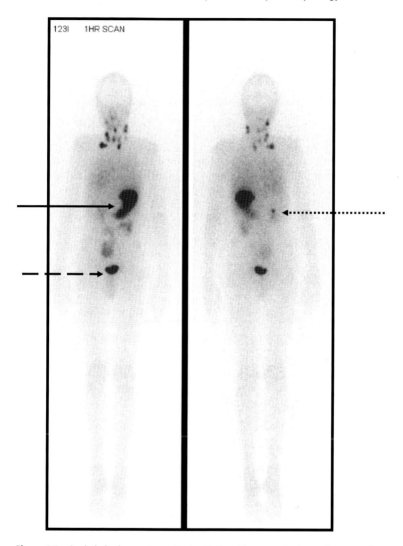

Figure 2.2. A whole-body scan in a patient with thyroid cancer who has undergone a thyroidectomy. The scan shows trapping of iodine in lymph node metastases within 1 hour of ingestion of an oral dose of [123]I. There is still activity in the stomach and the urinary tract and bladder demonstrate excretion of the radioactivity.

for formation of new thyroid hormones. Tg can be measured in the serum of normal people (range of <0.5–50 ng/mL). Serum Tg is a marker for residual thyroid cancer when the thyroid has been removed surgically.

Carriage of Thyroid Hormones in the Blood

Thyroid hormones are released into the circulation where 0.03% T_4 and 0.3% of T_3 are free, the remainder being protein bound. The unbound or free hormone is the active component. Thyroid binding globulin, transthyretin, and albumin are the main thyroid transporters. They provide a buffer so that sudden changes in hormone can be modulated.

Metabolism of Thyroid Hormones

Thyroid hormones are metabolized by deiodination. Eighty to ninety percent of T_3 is produced by deiodination of T_4 in peripheral tissues. Thyroid hormone can be metabolized by conjugation with glucuronide or sulfate in the liver and can be identified on posttherapy scans after a patient with thyroid cancer has been treated with a large dose of ^{131}I. A small proportion of thyroid hormones are degraded by deamination and decarboxylation of the amino terminal of the molecule.

Action of Thyroid Hormones

The main actions of thyroid hormones are genomic. There are also effects on mitochondria and cell membranes. T_3 attaches to specific thyroid hormone receptors within the nucleus. Each receptor has a central domain for binding to DNA, and a region at the carboxyl terminal for binding T_3 and for controlling transcription. Nongenomic actions of thyroid hormones have been described on the plasma membrane, mitochondria, cytoplasm, and cytoskeleton.

Effects of Thyroid Hormones on the Individual

One aspect of treatment of patients with thyroid cancer involves withdrawing thyroid hormone to produce clinical and biochemical hypothyroidism. Over the course of 4 weeks without thyroid hormones, patients gain weight, become tired and depressed, their skin dries and wrinkles, their hair loses luster, and they become constipated, cold, and miserable. The deprivation and replacement of thyroid hormone allows us to witness the many functions of thyroid hormones on virtually all the tissues of the body. In contrast, at times a supraphysiologic dose of thyroid hormone is prescribed and the symptoms and sign of mild thyrotoxicosis can be diagnosed.

Control of Thyroid Function: Hypothalamic-Pituitary-Thyroid Axis

The anterior pituitary secretes the glycoprotein TSH. The pituitary is controlled positively by thyrotropin-releasing hormone (TRH) and negatively by thyroid hormones. TRH is synthesized and secreted in the paraventricular nuclei of the hypothalamus. TRH is a tripeptide: glutamyl-histidyl-prolinamide and it stimulates formation and secretion of TSH. TRH receptor is a G protein–coupled 7 transmembrane receptor. TRH increases several steps of TSH synthesis and secretion, in particular the control of the posttranslational maturation of TSH oligosaccharide chains.[6] In the absence of TRH, TSH lacks its full biologic activity. TRH and thyroid hormones have a complex interaction. The expression of the thyroid hormone receptor in the thyrotroph is lowered by TRH, thus reducing the negative feedback of T_3. Historically, the intravenous injection of TRH was a valuable test to diagnose mild thyrotoxicosis. The production of the only FDA-approved preparation in the United States has recently stopped. TRH is metabolized by an enzyme called TRH-degrading ectoenzyme.[7] TRH is present in other parts of the brain and has a putative role as a neurotransmitter. TRH has been used to treat neurologic conditions and epilepsy.[8] It has been shown to reduce the intake of food in experimental animals.[9]

Pituitary and Thyroid-Stimulating Hormone

TSH is a glycoprotein containing two peptide chains, α and β.[10] The α peptide is common to luteinizing hormone, follicle-stimulating hormone, and human chorionic gonadotropin. The β subunit of each of these hormones is different and confers specific biologic and immunologic function. In the case of TSH, the β peptide is only produced in thyrotrophs that constitute about 5% of the cells in the anterior pituitary. The α chain contains 92 amino acids and is encoded by a gene on chromosome 6. The β subunit has 112 amino acids and is encoded by a gene on chromosome 1. The posttranslational attachment of sugar molecules is important for full function. TSH lacking sugars can bind to the TSH receptor but has reduced function.

Serum TSH can be measured precisely and is the single, most important test of thyroid function (see below). TSH increases all steps of thyroid hormone production including trapping of iodine and iodination of tyrosine. An increased TSH is important in testing and treating patients who have had thyroidectomy for thyroid cancer and who are to undergo scintiscan or treatment with radionuclides of iodine or measurement of a stimulated Tg. A high level of TSH is achieved by letting the patient become hypothyroid, but patients do not like the symptoms of hypothyroidism. Recombinant human TSH can be used for testing and treating patients and is described in detail in Chapter 5.[11,12]

There is evidence that a number of proteins are local "autocrine/ paracrine" regulators of TSH secretion.[13] Epidermal growth factor has a positive effect and neurotensin, neuromedin B, interleukin-1, and gastrin-releasing peptide have inhibitory roles. These are considerably less important than the positive TRH action and the negative feedback of thyroid hormones. T_3 attached to its specific receptor in thyrotrophs has an inhibitory action on the gene that transcribes mRNA of TSH β. This is the key in negative feedback.

TSH Receptor

The TSH receptor is a G protein–coupled receptor. The gene is on chromosome 14q31. The receptor has a large extracellular domain with a tertiary structure that is important for binding with TSH. In the presence of TSH, there is increased production of intracellular cyclic adenosine monophosphate (cAMP). This occurs through the receptor interacting with the G_s complex and causing disassociation of the α subunit from the β and γ subunits. The α subunit is complexed with guanosine diphosphate (GDP) and it releases the GDP, which is replaced by guanosine triphosphate. This compound activates the enzyme adenyl cyclase converting adenosine 5'-triphosphate to cAMP. With the increase in intracellular cAMP, there is an increased uptake of iodine, production of TPO and Tg, and release of thyroid hormones. Prolonged TSH stimulation produces growth of follicular cells. When the concentration of TSH is high, the calcium phosphatidyl-inositol-phosphate protein kinase pathway is activated and this increases production of H_2O_2.

A number of mutations have been identified in the TSH receptor. Some of these produce a gain in function. When the activating mutation is on a clone of thyroid cells (a somatic mutation), this results in a functioning nodule or functioning nodular goiter. A germ line mutation affecting all follicular cells causes a rare form of neonatal thyrotoxicosis that should be differentiated from neonatal Graves' disease. There are also mutations that inactivate the TSH receptor causing a resistance to TSH. Activating mutations in the G_s α subunit can produce the same effects as activating mutations of the TSH receptor.

TSH increases the formation and release of thyroid hormones resulting in an increase in free T_4 (and or free T_3) that in turn produces the negative feedback at the level of the thyrotroph and to a lesser extent the hypothalamus.

Autoregulation of the Thyroid

Iodine has autoregulatory effects on the thyroid with the goal of maintaining a steady physiologic state. The use of inorganic iodine to reduce the thyrotoxic effects of Graves' disease demonstrates this. High levels of iodine reduce its own transport into follicular cells also reducing its organification (Wolff-Chaikoff effect).[14] When the intake of iodine is chronically reduced, the thyroid produces a higher ratio of T_3/T_4. This provides the more active hormone at the expense of less iodine (T_3 has three fourths of the iodine and about 4 times the activity so there is more than $5:1$ benefit).

Testing Thyroid Function

The best tests to determine thyroid function are FT_4 and TSH. It is true that testing thyroid function in outpatients who have a high probability of being normal can be achieved by measurement of TSH alone.[15] In patients with thyroid cancer, the clinician can titrate the dose of thyroid hormone to the desired level of TSH for each individual patient. There have been progressive increases in sensitivity of the assays resulting in a lowering of the level of detectability for TSH and most can now achieve functional sensitivities of <0.005 mIU/L. An extensive monograph of practice guidelines for laboratory testing of thyroid function is available.[16]

Thyroid scintigraphy and uptake measurement using ^{123}I have a limited role in the management of patients with a newly diagnosed thyroid nodule but would be ordered when thyroid function is high. Whole-body scan with ^{131}I or ^{123}I is used in many patients with differentiated thyroid cancer to define how much thyroid has been left after thyroidectomy and to identify functioning metastases. An uptake measurement obtained over the thyroid bed and sites of cancer at the time of scanning provides a quantification of the amount of functioning thyroid.

Tg can be measured accurately by radioimmunoassays and immunoradiometric assays. This measurement is very important in the management of patients with thyroid cancer who have been treated. The Tg value should be undetectable or low (normal 0.5–50.0 ng/mL).

Calcitonin secreted by parafollicular C cells and normal values are usually <10 ng/L (10 pg/mL). This measurement is important in follow-up of patients with medullary cancer.

References

1. Peretz A, Leiberman E, Kapelushnik J, Hershkovitz E. Thyroglossal duct carcinoma in children: case presentation and review of the literature. Thyroid 2004;14(9): 777–785.

2. Schmutzler C. Regulation of the sodium/iodide symporter by retinoids—a review. Exp Clin Endocrinol Diabetes 2001;109(1):41–44.

3. Darcan S, Goksen D. Consequences of iodine deficiency and preventative measures. Pediatric Endocrine Rev 2003;1:162–168.

4. Levy O, De la Vieja A, Carrasco N. The Na+/I– symporter (NIS): recent advances. J Bioenerg Biomembr 1998;30(2):195–206.

5. Russo D, Manole D, Arturi F, et al. Absence of sodium/iodide symporter gene mutations in differentiated human thyroid carcinomas. Thyroid 2001;11(1):37–39.

6. Persani L. Hypothalamic thyrotropin-releasing hormone and thyrotropin biological activity. Thyroid 1998;8:941–946.

7. Heuer H, Schafer MK, Bauer K. Thyrotropin-releasing hormone (TRH), a signal peptide of the central nervous system. Acta Med Austriaca 1999;26:119–122.

8. Zervas IM, Papakostas YG, Theodoropoulou MA, Dimitrakopoulos C, Vaidakis N, Daras M. Thyrotropin-releasing hormone administration does not affect seizure threshold during electroconvulsive therapy. J Ect 2003;19(3):136–138.

9. Choi YH, Hartzell D, Azain MJ, Baile CA. TRH decreases food intake and increases water intake and body temperature in rats. Physiol Behav 2002;77(1):1–4.

10. Szkudlinski MW, Fremont V, Ronin C, Weintraub BD. Thyroid-stimulating hormone and thyroid-stimulating hormone receptor structure-function relationships. Physiol Rev 2002;82(2):473–502.

11. Joshi L, Murata Y, Wondisford FE, Szkudlinski MW, Desai R, Weintraub BD. Recombinant thyrotropin containing a beta-subunit chimera with the human chorionic gonadotropin-beta carboxy-terminus is biologically active, with a prolonged plasma half-life: role of carbohydrate in bioactivity and metabolic clearance. Endocrinology 1995;136(9):3839–3848.

12. Szkudlinski MW, Thotakura NR, Bucci I, et al. Purification and characterization of recombinant human thyrotropin (TSH) isoforms produced by Chinese hamster ovary cells: the role of sialylation and sulfation in TSH bioactivity. Endocrinology 1993;133(4):1490–1503.

13. Pazos-Moura CC, Ortiga-Carvalho TM, Gaspar de Moura E. The autocrine/paracrine regulation of thyrotropin secretion. Thyroid 2003;13(2):167–175.

14. Berkowitz M, Daughtridge D, Sherwin JR. Autoregulation of thyroid iodide transport: possible mediation by modification in sodium cotransport. Am J Physiol 1981;240(1):E37–42.

15. Viera AJ. Thyroid function testing in outpatients: are both sensitive thyrotropin (sTSH) and free thyroxine (FT4) necessary? Fam Med 2003;35(6):408–410.

16. Demers LM, Spencer CA. Laboratory medicine practice guidelines: laboratory support for the diagnosis and monitoring of thyroid disease. Clin Endocrinol (Oxf) 2003;58(2):138–140.

3. Thyroid Nodule

In the United States (US), 4%–7% of adults, predominately women, have a palpable thyroid nodule. At autopsy, thyroid nodules are found in about 50% of adults. Nodules are noted in approximately 30%–50% on ultrasound or computed tomography of the thyroid. It is important to differentiate the rare cancerous thyroid nodule from the large proportion that is benign. Impalpable nodules picked up on imaging studies are called incidentalomas.[1] Causes of a benign nodule include colloid nodule, adenoma, adenomatous goiter, cysts, cystic degeneration of a preexisting nodule, autoimmune thyroid disease such as Hashimoto's, and subacute thyroiditis. Management involves attention to clinical features, biochemical tests, and additional investigations, in particular fine needle aspiration (FNA).

Clinical Features

Thyroid nodules are usually asymptomatic and most frequently the nodule is identified during a physical examination. A large nodule causes symptoms such as pressure, difficulty swallowing and or breathing, and a change in voice. Pain in a thyroid nodule is uncommon and is caused either by bleeding into a nodule or subacute thyroiditis. Pain from a thyroid abscess (acute thyroiditis), or rapidly growing cancer such as lymphoma and anaplastic cancer, is very uncommon. Some clinical features increase the risk of a nodule being malignant (Table 3.1). These include young and old age, male gender, family history of thyroid cancer, and prior radiation over the neck. Cancerous nodules are more likely to be hard, irregular, and fixed to adjacent structures. However, history and clinical examination cannot differentiate most thyroid cancers from benign nodules.

Diagnostic Testing

The optimal test in a euthyroid patient is FNA of the nodule with cytopathologic interpretation of the aspirated cells (Figure 3.1). Most patients with a malignant thyroid nodule are clinically and biochemically euthyroid. This is confirmed by normal levels of thyrotropin (TSH) and free thyroxine. A thyroid nodule in a hyperthyroid patient can be the result of an autonomous nodule producing an excess of thyroid hormones or Graves' disease with a nonfunctioning nodule. [123]I scintiscan is the best first test in a hyperthyroid patient.

Table 3.1. Clinical features that increase the possibility of a malignant versus a benign thyroid nodule

Malignant	Benign	Evidence and discussion
Patient age <20 years Patient age >60 years	More likely between 20 and 60 years	Cancer is most common in 30–50 age range but there is an even higher incidence of benign nodules in this age range.
Man	Woman	This seems paradoxical because thyroid cancer is more common in women (3 : 1) but benign nodules are less common in men.
Nodule single	Multiple nodules	Note that thyroid cancer can occur in multinodular goiter.
Nodule hard	Nodule soft	
Nodule fixed	Nodule mobile	
Nodule irregular	Nodule smooth	
Nodule painless	Nodule painful	Painful lesions are rare, include thyroiditis and bleeding into nodule. Carcinomatous pseudothyroiditis is very rare.
Rapid growth of nodule	Slow growth	However, most thyroid cancers are slow-growing
Invasive Recurrent laryngeal nerve Esophagus Trachea Soft tissues	No invasion	
Lymph node metastases	No lymph node metastases	This confirms malignancy.
Distant metastases Lung Bone Brain Soft tissues	No distant metastases	This confirms malignancy.
Familial thyroid cancer Medullary including MEN syndromes Nonmedullary familial thyroid cancer	No familial thyroid cancer	Familial differentiated thyroid cancer is being recognized more often.

Source: Adapted from McDougall.[32]
MEN, multiple endocrine neoplasia.

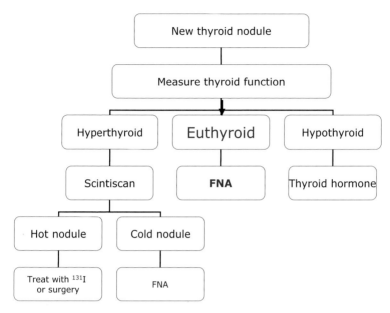

Figure 3.1. An algorithm for evaluation of a thyroid nodule. (From McDougall.[32])

An autonomous nodule called a "hot" nodule because of its appearance on scintiscan is almost always benign and FNA is not necessary. A nonfunctioning nodule in Graves' disease can be benign or malignant and an FNA of the lesion is important. A higher incidence of cancer has been reported in nonfunctioning nodules in Graves' disease. When the patient is hypothyroid and has a nodule, the diagnosis includes Hashimoto's thyroiditis and thyroid hormone might cause the nodule to shrink. Should the nodule not diminish in size after 3–6 months of L-thyroxine, it should be biopsied.

Thyroid Scintigraphy

Thyroid scintigraphy is frequently ordered by primary care physicians who believe that the test can help differentiate a benign from a malignant thyroid nodule. The belief is that nonfunctioning "cold" nodules have a high probability of being malignant. This is not true. In a metaanalysis, Ashcraft and Van Herle[2] found the specificity of scintigraphy to be 15%. When the patient is hyperthyroid, the most appropriate radionuclide for scintigraphy is [123]I. I obtain a 24-hour uptake and scan after 200–300μCi (7.4–11.1 MBq).

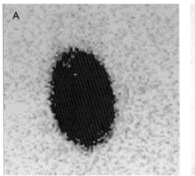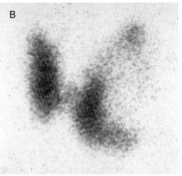

Figure 3.2. A ^{123}I scintiscan shows a functioning nodule with complete suppression of the uptake in the remainder of the normal thyroid. **B** A nonfunctioning nodule in the left lobe of the thyroid.

^{99m}TcO$_4$ is also used for imaging; it is trapped but not organified. Scans and quantitative measurements of ^{99m}TcO$_4$ are made 10–20 minutes after the intravenous injection of that radiopharmaceutical. A proportion of nodules that are "hot" on ^{99m}TcO$_4$ scan are "cold" using ^{123}I. This increases the probability of cancer and supports my preference for ^{123}I. It has been emphasized that autonomous functioning nodules in adults are usually benign. Figure 3.2 shows a typical functioning "hot" and nonfunctioning "cold" nodule. Most images are obtained with a pin-hole collimator but some authorities recommend single photon emission computed tomography, which improves resolution from 15 mm for planar imaging to 6–7 mm.[3]

Cancer-seeking radiopharmaceuticals such as thallium (^{201}Tl), ^{99m}Tc-sestamibi, and ^{99m}Tc-tetrafosmin do not help. There are a few reports of positron emission tomography differentiating benign from malignant thyroid nodules but the numbers of patients studied are small and the incomplete separation of cancerous nodules from benign are not encouraging.

Thyroid Ultrasound

Ultrasound cannot clearly differentiate a benign from malignant nodule. It is used for follow-up evaluation of size and characteristics of nodules. Nodules surrounded by a "halo" are likely to be benign and a "comet tail" appearance is a reliable indicator of abundant colloid, which usually indicates a benign colloid nodule.[4] Cancers are likely to be solid and hypoechoic and have microcalcifications.[5]

Fine Needle Aspiration

FNA is highly sensitive and specific.[6,7] It is the best and most cost-effective test to determine whether a nodule is cancerous or not.[8,9] It also has a role in children. FNA specimens are usually reported as A) benign, B) cancer or suspicious for cancer, C) indeterminate, and D) nondiagnostic or inadequate. When there are insufficient cells, the procedure should be repeated using ultrasound guidance. Ultrasound also allows small, difficult to feel and even impalpable nodules to be sampled. Repeat biopsy of a proven benign nodule is not very helpful because the second study usually shows the same features of a benign thyroid.[10] FNA and ultrasound are increasingly accepted as complementary.

Management of Thyroid Nodule

FNA is the central investigation (Figure 3.1). When the thyroid nodule is malignant, the patient should be referred for thyroidectomy. When it is benign, the patient can be reassured but there must be continuity of care. When the FNA is indeterminate, there is a 10%–20% chance of cancer. The cytopathology demonstrates a microfollicular pattern with small amounts of colloid and it is not possible to exclude follicular cancer, or follicular variant of papillary cancer, without histology.[11] Most thyroid physicians would refer the patient for operation. Male gender, a solitary nodule larger than 4 cm, and a family history of thyroid cancer increase the risk of a lesion being cancer.

Treatment with Thyroid Hormone

In a controlled study, patients with benign colloid nodules were treated with thyroid hormone, or placebo for 6 months and then the medications were switched.[12] There was no statistical difference in nodule size measured by ultrasound. A metaanalysis showed no statistical benefit but there was a "trend towards a reduction" in nodule size.[13] Potential complications of long-term low TSH include loss of bone mass, increase in cardiac arrhythmias, and behavioral irregularities. In the US, thyroid hormone is usually not prescribed to euthyroid patients with a benign thyroid nodule.

Treatment of Autonomous Thyroid Nodule Causing Thyrotoxicosis

A hyperfunctioning nodule can be treated by lobectomy, radioiodine ^{131}I, or by injection of ethanol. Antithyroid medications can be administered with the goal of controlling thyrotoxicosis before proceeding with definitive therapy or in a very old patient whose life expectancy is short. Larger nodules and younger patients are usually treated by operation. [131]I is preferred for older patients.

Cystic Thyroid Nodule

A cystic nodule can be monitored clinically and by ultrasound. It can be aspirated and if it recurs, it can be observed, drained again, injected with sclerosant, or removed.

Management of Multinodular Goiter

The first step is to determine if the patient is hyperthyroid, euthyroid, or hypothyroid. In hyperthyroid patients, a scintiscan demonstrates whether there are multiple functioning nodules or nodules superimposed on Graves' disease (Marine-Lenhart syndrome). Toxic multinodular goiter can be treated by surgery or ^{131}I, and the specific choice is based on age of the patient, size of the goiter, personal preference of the patient, and availability of trained specialists. Nygaard et al.[14] on review of their results using ^{131}I in 130 patients with toxic nodular goiter conclude, "Ninety-two percent of patients with multinodular toxic goiter were cured with 1 or 2 treatments. The thyroid volume was reduced by 43%, with few side effects. Iodine 131 should be the choice of treatment in patients with multinodular toxic goiter." A hypothetical reason for not treating with radioiodine is swelling of the goiter and worsening of pressure effects after [131]I. This has been shown to be a myth by ultrasound measurements of thyroid volume 2, 7, 14, 21, 28, and 35 days after therapy in 30 patients, some with toxic nodular goiter and some with nontoxic nodular goiter.[14]

In a euthyroid patient living in a region of iodine deficiency, supplemental iodine can have an effect in reducing goiter size. Monitoring of the thyroid size and function is important and some patients can develop Jod-Basedow phenomenon (iodine-induced thyrotoxicosis). A nodular goiter with normal thyroid function in a person who has lived in an iodine-replete country will not benefit from iodine. The options are to watch, to operate, or to treat with [131]I. An investigation in Australia presented a hypothetical patient to endocrine surgeons and endocrinologists. The patient was a 42-year-old woman with a 50- to 80-g multinodular goiter and normal thyroid function.[15] A majority of both the endocrinologists and surgeons advised no treatment (65% and 67%, respectively). The remainder of the endocrinologists recommended L-thyroxine (22%), surgery (10%), or [131]I (3%). For the surgeons, 31% recommended surgery and 2% L-thyroxine. The investigators provided 11 variations on the index patient and after analysis of responses concluded, "There are clinically significant differences between endocrine surgeons and endocrinologists in the management of multinodular goiter." When experts give different opinions, there is probably no one correct answer. An asymptomatic goiter can be left untreated but a nodular goiter that is causing pressure symptoms should be treated, and in the US, the common approach is by operation. This immediately corrects the symptoms and the patient takes replacement L-thyroxine for life. The complications of thyroidectomy including hematoma, damage to the recurrent and external laryngeal nerves, and parathyroids are not common when the operation is conducted by a well-trained, experienced surgeon. Treatment with radioiodine is less attractive because the uptake by the goiter is usually low and this coupled with the size of the gland mean that a very large dose of ^{131}I has to be administered. In addition, the reduction in size is not great and it takes several months to achieve that. Nygaard et al. treated 69 patients with 3.7 MBq/g (100 μCi/g) corrected for uptake. Fifty-six patients received one treatment, one patient had four therapies, and the remainder two. Comparison of thyroid volume in 39 patients before and 24 months after therapy showed a reduction from 73 to 29 mL. Eleven percent became hypothyroid. The results are impressive but it is hard to understand how such small administered doses can have such a great effect.

Graves' disease has developed in a few patients after radioiodine treatment of both toxic and nontoxic nodular goiter.[16,17] This is probably attributable to formation of thyroid-stimulating antibodies in response to the release of thyroid antigens. Several authorities recommend ^{131}I as the treatment of choice in the elderly.[18-20] Nevertheless, a large goiter size and low uptake make the treatment inappropriate for some patients. I have not been impressed with the results in patients I have treated, but the selection of patients could be a factor.[21]

Recombinant human TSH (rhTSH) is approved for increasing the uptake in thyroid cancer. This is discussed in detail in Chapter 5. There are several reports of rhTSH to increase the uptake in nodular goiter as a preliminary to ^{131}I treatment. Twenty-two patients were treated with radioiodine after 0.01– 0.03 mg of rhTSH.[22] The uptake doubled, therefore the therapy dose was reduced by a factor of 2. There was a reduction in goiter size of about 40%. Duick and Baskin[23] treated 16 patients with 1.1 GBq (30 mCi) after 0.9 mg of rhTSH was administered to 10 patients and 0.3 mg of rhTSH to 6 patients. The uptakes increased by a factor of 4. Some were biochemically hyperthyroid before treatment with ^{131}I and in all cases TSH became normal or increased above normal after ^{131}I treatment. The authors estimated a 30%–40% reduction in goiter size over 3–7 months and there was symptomatic improvement.

L-Thyroxine should be prescribed for patients with goiter who are biochemically hypothyroid. This treatment is ineffective for euthyroid nodular goiter.[24] It can be dangerous for patients with toxic nodular goiter. Once the patient has been euthyroid for months and the goiter has failed to shrink, it is advisable to refer for surgery.

A problem is the recurrence of nontoxic nodular goiter after surgery. This generally is the result of the surgeon leaving too much tissue or conducting a lobectomy. When the recurrent goiter is symptomatic, the therapies are surgery or [131]I. Repeat thyroid operations are associated with a higher incidence of complications and should be undertaken by an experienced operator who has conducted "redo" procedures. An alternative that has been used in Europe is injection of the nodules with ethanol.[25]

Substernal (Retrosternal) Nodular Goiter

Substernal goiter is more common in goitrous regions and in older people. To be defined as substernal, 50% or more of the goiter should be intrathoracic. Many cases are identified by an X-ray or computed tomography scan obtained for a nonthyroidal reason but when the diagnosis is established and patients questioned directly the majority have noted a change in breathing. The goiter can cause compression on adjacent structures and can be the cause of tracheal compression, superior vena cava syndrome, recurrent laryngeal nerve paralysis, difficulty in swallowing, and even chylothorax.[26] [123]I scintiscan confirms that there is thyroid present ($^{99m}TcO_4$ is not advised). The uptake of radioiodine is frequently patchy except in the rare case of thyrotoxicosis in the substernal goiter.[27] FNA of retrosternal goiter is not recommended because of the proximity of the great vessel. Surgery is usually recommended.[28] The general health of the patient is important, and in the elderly or frail when there is high uptake of a tracer of radioiodine, ^{131}I can be considered.[29] This produces about 30% reduction in volume.[30] In one report, 158 of 170 were excised through a standard collar incision.[28] Permanent damage to the parathyroids and recurrent laryngeal nerves is rare. The incidence of cancer in surgically removed glands ranges from 2.5% to 13% and thus mirrors the range for nodular glands in the cervical position.[28,31]

Summary and Key Facts

Solitary thyroid nodules and nodular goiter are common. Most patients are euthyroid and the best investigation is FNA of the nodule or dominant nodule. A scintiscan is a valuable first investigation in thyrotoxic patients because an autonomous "hot" nodule in an adult has minimal risk of being a cancer and can be treated by lobectomy or [131]I (or injection with ethanol).

References

1. Topliss D. Thyroid incidentaloma: the ignorant in pursuit of the impalpable. Clin Endocrinol (Oxf) 2004;60(1):18–20.
2. Ashcraft M, Van Herle AJ. Management of the thyroid nodule. Scanning techniques, thyroid suppressive therapy and fine-needle aspiration. Head Neck Surg 1981; 3:297–322.

3. Wanet P, Sand A, Abramovici J. Physical and clinical evaluation of high-resolution thyroid pinhole tomography. J Nucl Med 1996;37:2017–2020.

4. Ahuja A, Chick W, King W, Metreweli C. Clinical significance of the comet-tail artifact in thyroid ultrasound. J Clin Ultrasound 1996;24(3):129–133.

5. Chan BK, Desser TS, McDougall IR, Weigel RJ, Jeffrey RB Jr. Common and uncommon sonographic features of papillary thyroid carcinoma. J Ultrasound Med 2003; 22(10):1083–1090.

6. Afroze N, Kayani N, Hasan SH. Role of fine needle aspiration cytology in the diagnosis of palpable thyroid lesions. Indian J Pathol Microbiol 2002;45(3): 241–246.

7. Agrawal S. Diagnostic accuracy and role of fine needle aspiration cytology in management of thyroid nodules. J Surg Oncol 1995;58(3):168–172.

8. Solomon D, Keeler EB. Cost-effective analysis of the evaluation of thyroid nodule. Ann Intern Med 1982;96:221–232.

9. Singer PA. Thyroid nodules: malignant or benign? Hosp Pract (Minneap) 1998; 33(1):143–144, 147–148, 153–156.

10. Aguilar J, Rodriguez JM, Flores B, et al. Value of repeated fine-needle aspiration cytology and cytologic experience on the management of thyroid nodules. Otolaryngol Head Neck Surg 1998;119(1):121–124.

11. Logani S, Osei SY, LiVolsi VA, Baloch ZW. Fine-needle aspiration of follicular variant of papillary carcinoma in a hyperfunctioning thyroid nodule. Diagn Cytopathol 2001;25(1):80–81.

12. Gharib H, James EM, Charboneau JW, Naessens JM, Offord KP, Gorman CA. Suppressive therapy with levothyroxine for solitary thyroid nodules. A double-blind controlled clinical study. N Engl J Med 1987;317:70–75.

13. Castro MR, Caraballo PJ, Morris JC. Effectiveness of thyroid hormone suppressive therapy in benign solitary thyroid nodules: a meta-analysis. J Clin Endocrinol Metab 2002;87(9):4154–4159.

14. Nygaard B, Faber J, Hegedus L. Acute changes in thyroid volume and function following 131I therapy of multinodular goitre. Clin Endocrinol (Oxf) 1994;41(6): 715–718.

15. Bhagat MC, Dhaliwal SS, Bonnema SJ, Hegedus L, Walsh JP. Differences between endocrine surgeons and endocrinologists in the management of non-toxic multinodular goitre. Br J Surg 2003;90(9):1103–1112.

16. Nygaard B, Faber J, Veje A, Hegedus L, Hansen JM. Appearance of Graves'-like disease after radioiodine therapy for toxic as well as non-toxic multinodular goitre. Clin Endocrinol (Oxf) 1995;43(1):129–130.

17. Chiovato L, Santini F, Vitti P, Bendinelli G, Pinchera A. Appearance of thyroid stimulating antibody and Graves' disease after radioiodine therapy for toxic nodular goitre. Clin Endocrinol (Oxf) 1994;40(6):803–806.

18. Verelst J, Bonnyns M, Glinoer D. Radioiodine therapy in voluminous multinodular non-toxic goitre. Acta Endocrinol (Copenh) 1990;122(4):417–421.

19. Manders JM, Corstens FH. Radioiodine therapy of euthyroid multinodular goitres. Eur J Nucl Med Mol Imaging 2002;29(suppl 2):S466–470.

20. Glinoer D. Radioiodine therapy of non-toxic multinodular goitre. Clin Endocrinol (Oxf) 1994;41(6):713–714.

21. Hartoft-Nielsen ML, Rasmussen AK, Friis E, et al. Unsuccessful radioiodine treatment of a non-toxic goiter: a case report. Basic Clin Pharmacol Toxicol 2004; 95(2):72–75.

22. Nieuwlaat WA, Huysmans DA, van den Bosch HC, et al. Pretreatment with a single, low dose of recombinant human thyrotropin allows dose reduction of radioiodine therapy in patients with nodular goiter. J Clin Endocrinol Metab 2003;88(7): 3121–3129.

23. Duick DS, Baskin HJ. Utility of recombinant human thyrotropin for augmentation of radioiodine uptake and treatment of nontoxic and toxic multinodular goiters. Endocr Pract 2003;9(3):204–209.

24. Hegedus L, Bonnema SJ, Bennedbaek FN. Management of simple nodular goiter: current status and future perspectives. Endocr Rev 2003;24(1):102–132.

25. Solymosi T, Gal I. Treatment of recurrent nodular goiters with percutaneous ethanol injection: a clinical study of twelve patients. Thyroid 2003;13(3):273–277.

26. Villanueva R, Haber R. Tracheal compression in a patient with substernal extension of a multinodular goiter. Thyroid 2000;10(4):367.

27. Fogelfeld L, Rubinstein U, Bar-On J, Feigl D. Severe thyrotoxicosis caused by an ectopic intrathoracic goiter. Clin Nucl Med 1986;11(1):20–22.

28. Erbil Y, Bozbora A, Barbaros U, Ozarmagan S, Azezli A, Molvalilar S. Surgical management of substernal goiters: clinical experience of 170 cases. Surg Today 2004; 34(9):732–736.

29. Drivas I, Mansberg R, Roberts JM, Kean AM. Massive intrathoracic toxic multinodular goiter treated with radioiodine. Clin Nucl Med 2003;28(2):138–139.

30. Bonnema SJ, Knudsen DU, Bertelsen H, et al. Does radioiodine therapy have an equal effect on substernal and cervical goiter volumes? Evaluation by magnetic resonance imaging. Thyroid 2002;12(4):313–317.

31. Katlic MR, Grillo HC, Wang CA. Substernal goiter. Analysis of 80 patients from Massachusetts General Hospital. Am J Surg 1985;149(2):283–287.

32. McDougall I. Management of Thyroid Cancer and Related Nodular Disease. London: Springer-Verlag; 2006:95–133.

4. Thyroid Pathology*

Cancers that arise from follicular cells are classified along a morphologic spectrum into well-differentiated carcinomas at one pole and anaplastic (undifferentiated) carcinomas at the other. Well-differentiated carcinomas retain the appearance of follicular cells and can trap iodine and secrete thyroglobulin (Tg). Based on histology, they are subclassified as papillary, or follicular types. Anaplastic carcinomas are undifferentiated neoplasms of follicular cell origin that often bear little resemblance to follicular cells. C cells (parafollicular cells) can undergo malignant transformation and are called medullary cancer. Lymphomas and leukemias arise from hematolymphoid cells and sarcomas are of mesenchymal cell origin. In geographic regions of high iodine intake, about 80% of thyroid cancers are differentiated and, of these, 90% are papillary carcinomas, 5%–10% follicular carcinomas, another 5%–10% are medullary carcinomas, 2%–5% anaplastic carcinomas, and 2%–5% malignant lymphomas (Figure 4.1). Rarely, nonthyroidal cancers can metastasize to the thyroid. A close working relationship with a pathologist interested in thyroid pathology is indispensable in the management of patients, and pathology slides of patients referred for treatment from another institution should always be reviewed. Treatment and prognosis are determined in large part by the histologic type of neoplasm. For example, it is essential that adenoma be carefully distinguished from minimally invasive or widely invasive follicular carcinoma. This chapter discusses both cytologic findings of fine needle aspiration (FNA) specimens and the histologic features of inflammatory and neoplastic conditions.

Fine Needle Aspiration

The principal role of FNA is to provide the accurate pathologic diagnosis and classification of a thyroid nodule. Five diagnostic categories are used: malignant, suspicious for malignancy, indeterminate, benign, and inadequate. In general, the first three warrant a surgical biopsy for histopathologic confirmation. Many authors require the presence of at least 6 clusters of 10–20 cells on each of 1–2 slides for specimen adequacy. Nayar and Frost[1] emphasize three steps in the analysis of FNA: 1) the arrangement of cells with respect to one another, 2) the cytologic features of individual cells, and 3) the composition of background elements. Rapid smearing of the material for preparation of air-dried slides and alcohol-fixed slides is essential for preserving cytologic

---

*With special contribution from Gerald J. Berry

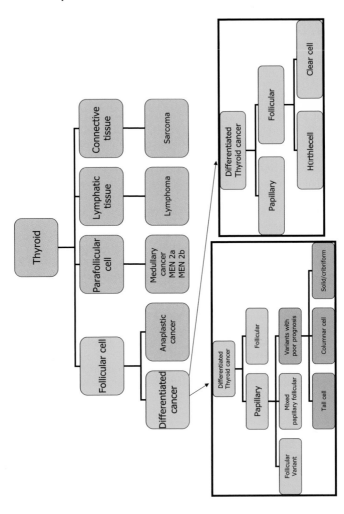

Figure 4.1. The algorithm illustrates the types of cancers found in the thyroid gland and their cell of origin.

detail. The amount and type of colloid should be included in the report. The size of follicles should be described and whether they are monotonous and microfollicular in arrangement. Nuclear features including size, grooves, and intranuclear pseudoinclusions are important for the diagnosis of papillary cancer. The techniques for FNA include FNA by palpation and ultrasound-guided FNA for nonpalpable lesions. In experienced hands (combining technical and diagnostic expertise), the false-negative rate is <5% and the false-positive rate is also low, around 1%–3%.[2]

Intraoperative Examination

Intraoperative evaluation by cytologic techniques and frozen section histology is used to determine whether an indeterminate lesion is malignant or to examine regional lymph nodes for metastases thus confirming cancer is present. Total thyroidectomy would then be undertaken. The distinction between follicular adenoma and minimally invasive well-differentiated carcinoma and their variants is seldom resolved on frozen section. On occasion, there can be a discrepancy between FNA and frozen section interpretation and some consider FNA to be more sensitive.[3]

Recent Molecular Advances

The use of specific labeled antibodies to stain tissue sections has increased the accuracy of histologic diagnosis.[4] These include Tg, galectin-3, calcitonin, cytokeratin-19, thyroid transcription factor-1 (TTF-1), HBME-1, estrogen receptor, cell adhesion molecule α and β integrins, CD44, CA125, α-1-antitrysin, and S100. Activating point mutations of the *RAS* protooncogenes occur in follicular adenomas and carcinomas, and anaplastic carcinomas but are uncommon in papillary carcinomas and Hürthle cell tumors. Inactivating point mutations of the *p53* tumor suppressor gene are very common in anaplastic thyroid carcinoma and have been reported with less frequency in poorly differentiated (insular) carcinoma.[5] Point mutations of *RET* protooncogene have recently been identified in both the sporadic and familial [non-MEN (multiple endocrine neoplasia], MEN 2A and 2B) forms of medullary carcinoma.

Benign Thyroid Tumors and Tumor-Like Nodules

There are many benign causes of clinical nodules in the thyroid including adenomatous (nodular) hyperplasia, adenoma, chronic lymphocytic thyroiditis, subacute thyroiditis, and colloid cyst. In FNA preparations, the follicular cells are uniform in size and shape and their nuclei are central and similar in size to those of a lymphocyte. In addition, there is often an admixture of groups of follicular cells and cells stripped of their cytoplasm ("naked nuclei") and colloid that ranges from a "watery" appearance, to "cracked glass" or the more classic tenacious material.

Nontoxic Multinodular Goiter/Adenomatous Hyperplasia

A goiter or an enlarged thyroid arises from a variety of causes including inherited enzyme deficiency, neoplasia, inflammation, or nutrient deficiency. In regions of iodine deficiency, multinodular or "endemic" goiters occur and are the most common global cause of thyroid enlargement. Women are more likely to be affected and multiparity and older age increase the prevalence. The histopathologic terms that are most often used for sporadic goiters are adenomatous or nodular hyperplasia, hyperplastic colloid nodule, or adenomatoid goiter. FNA displays the same constituents as the normal thyroid gland including abundant colloid, follicular cells, and there can be Hürthle cells and macrophages containing hemosiderin (Figure 4.2). The gland is enlarged and there are usually many nodules of varying size but there is no evidence of encapsulation or parenchymal invasion. Many follicles are large but there is variation in size and shape and there is abundant colloid.

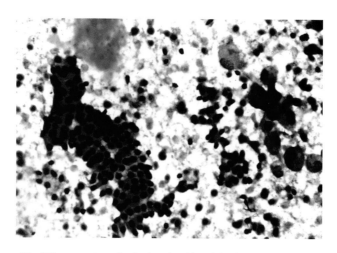

Figure 4.2. FNA preparation of a benign thyroid nodule showing bland follicular cells admixed with colloid and histiocytes (Diff-Quik ×400).

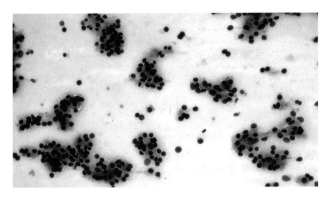

Figure 4.3. FNA findings of a follicular neoplasm demonstrating a repetitive microfollicular pattern and absence of colloid (Diff-Quik ×400).

Follicular Adenoma

Follicular adenoma is a solitary, encapsulated benign neoplasm of follicular cell origin that displays distinct differences in cellularity and composition from the adjacent normal thyroid parenchyma. The distinction of follicular adenoma from follicular carcinoma cannot reliably be made by FNA and the term "follicular neoplasm" is used. In FNA preparations, the smears are cellular with a repetitive array of microfollicles and scant colloid (Figure 4.3). Surgical excision is necessary to establish the correct histologic diagnosis. Follicular adenomas are solitary, round to oval, encapsulated, and smaller (1–3 cm in diameter) than nodular hyperplastic lesions (Figure 4.4). Hürthle cell adenomas are defined as benign tumors composed exclusively or predominantly (>75%) of oncocytic cells.[6] These large oxyphilic cells have a characteristic abundant red granular cytoplasm with round vesicular nuclei showing conspicuous central nucleoli in tissue sections. The abundance of mitochondria gives the cytoplasm its appearance. Capsular and vascular invasion is used to discriminate between benign and malignant lesions. The term "atypical follicular adenoma" is reserved for encapsulated neoplasms that according to the World Health Organization Committee display marked cellularity and unusual architectural and cytologic patterns such as necrosis or increased mitotic activity.[7] By definition, there should not be evidence of capsular or vascular invasion but the lesion has a worrisome appearance. In general, these have behaved in a benign manner. They must be distinguished from the recently coined term "follicular tumor of uncertain malignant potential," which is defined as a follicular neoplasm that shows incomplete or questionable penetration of the capsule.[8] It is thought that in some cases there is entrapment of tumor cells within the fibrous capsule or an irregular capsule.

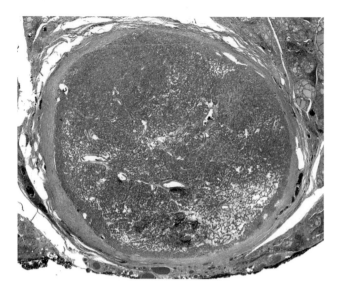

Figure 4.4. Low-power magnification of a follicular adenoma showing an encapsulated mass composed of follicular cells [hematoxylin and eosin (H&E) ×10].

Acute Thyroiditis (Thyroid Abscess)

Acute thyroiditis caused by bacterial or fungal infection is uncommon and this has been attributed to the high iodine content in the thyroid acting as an antiseptic. Most of the early reports were attributed to pyogenic bacterial organisms such as *Staphylococcus* sp., *Pneumococcus* sp., and *Streptococcus* sp.[9] Fungal organisms such as *Cryptococcus* sp., *Aspergillus* sp., and *Pneumocystis jiroveci* (formerly *P. carinii*) are reported in immunosuppressed patients.[10] FNA produces pus and necrotic debris. Histologically there are classic features of acute inflammatory exudates with abundant polymorphonuclear cells, necrosis, hemorrhage, and disruption of follicles.

Subacute Thyroiditis

Subacute thyroiditis or de Quervain's thyroiditis is a painful condition associated with systemic symptoms such as a viral illness plus thyrotoxicosis. FNA of the painful enlargement demonstrates multinucleated giant cells, inflammatory cells, and cellular debris admixed with degenerating follicular cells. Similar cells are seen on histopathologic sections, and the condition is also called "granulomatous thyroiditis." Other thyroid disorders that present with pain are acute thyroiditis, rarely Hashimoto's thyroiditis, and rapidly growing cancers causing pseudothyroiditis.[11] In general, painful conditions in the neck are more likely to be the result of nonthyroidal conditions such as laryngitis, pharyngitis, and esophagitis.

Chronic Lymphocytic Thyroiditis (Hashimoto's Thyroiditis)

Chronic lymphocytic thyroiditis or Hashimoto's thyroiditis is a very common organ-specific autoimmune disorder characterized by the presence of circulating antibodies against thyroid peroxidase (thyroid microsomal antigen) and Tg.[12] It is about 10 times more common in women, and an association with HLA-DR5 has been reported. FNA shows benign follicular cells and Hürthle cells admixed with inflammatory cells including small round lymphocytes, immunoblasts, tingible body macrophages, plasma cells, and occasionally multinucleated giant cells. Colloid is scanty or often absent. Microscopic sections reveal abundant lymphocytes and plasma cells, reactive germinal centers, and Hürthle cell metaplasia of follicles (Figure 4.5). The association of papillary cancer and Hashimoto's thyroiditis is well recognized and some authorities recommend careful search for any evidence of papillary cancer when the cytology is chronic lymphocytic thyroiditis.[13]

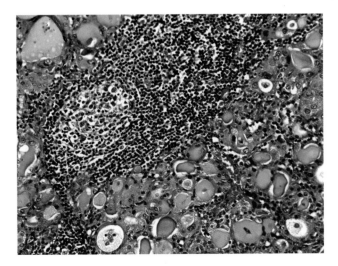

Figure 4.5. Hashimoto's thyroiditis composed of Hürthle cells and a reactive germinal center (H&E ×300).

Reidel's Thyroiditis

Reidel's thyroiditis is a rare inflammatory, sclerosing lesion of unknown etiology that can be associated with other fibrosing conditions such as retroperitoneal fibrosis, sclerosing cholangitis, mediastinal fibrosis, and orbital pseudotumor.[14] FNA usually yields scant fibrous material. The thyroid is enlarged, "woody" in consistency, and adherent to adjacent soft tissues. Histologically, the hallmark is dense sclerotic fibrous tissue with few follicular cells or colloid. The vessels show intimal proliferation, phlebitis, and intraluminal thrombi.

Thyroid Cancers

Differentiated Thyroid Cancer: Papillary Thyroid Cancer (Chapter 5)

In iodine sufficient regions, papillary cancer accounts for about 80%–90% of thyroid cancers. It is 3 times more common in women and the median age is 25–45 years. In cytologic preparations, there are avascular papillary fronds of cells showing crowding, nuclear enlargement, and metaplastic or "squamoid" cytoplasm. The nuclei might show grooves and pale inclusions (pseudoinclusions that are invaginations of cytoplasm) (Figure 4.6). The colloid often has a "bubble gum" appearance, and psammoma bodies and multinucleated giant cells are found in some cases. Papillary cancers are often bilateral and/or multifocal. The lesions are firm to hard and can have foci of calcification. The borders of these cancers are often irregular and infiltrative. Histologically, the cells are arranged in papillary fronds with central fibrovascular cores (Figure 4.7). The nuclei appear optically clear and have lateral displacement of the nucleoli near the nuclear membrane (so-called "Orphan Annie" nuclei after the comic strip character). Psammoma bodies are seen in about 50% of cases and derive from individual necrotic tumor cells that undergo calcification in lamellate layers. Lymphocytic response to the cancer cells is common. A minority of papillary cancers are solid or trabecular. Papillary cancers can contain areas of cystic degeneration. Papillary cancer spreads by lymphatics and involvement of regional nodes is common.

When papillary cancer is found serendipitously in a thyroid removed, for example a multinodular goiter and it is less than 1 cm, this is called an occult papillary cancer or microcarcinoma. This does not merit additional treatment.

Variants of Papillary Cancer (Chapter 6)

The follicular variant of papillary thyroid cancer is the most common. This can be difficult to diagnose in FNA samples. Histologically, the neoplasm is

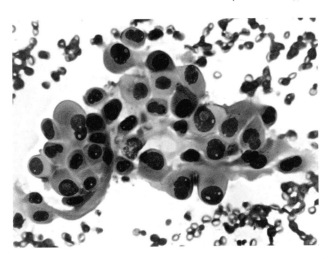

Figure 4.6. FNA findings in papillary carcinoma consisting of a papillary group without a central fibrovascular core, lined by enlarged cells with metaplastic "squamoid" cytoplasm with intranuclear pseudoinclusions (Diff-Quik ×600).

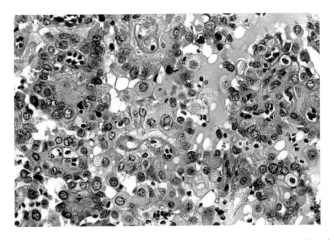

Figure 4.7. Histopathologic features of classic papillary carcinoma include papillary fronds lined by cells with intranuclear pseudoinclusions and nuclear grooves (H&E ×400).

composed of follicles lined by cells with the nuclear features of papillary cancer. The diffuse sclerosing variant is characterized by extensive replacement of one or both lobes by hyalinizing fibrous tissue and lymphoid cells. This pattern has been reported in 60%–70% of the children who developed papillary cancer after exposure to radiation in the Chernobyl reactor accident.

Tall cell and columnar cell variants have a worse prognosis. The height of the neoplastic cells is twice the width in the tall cell variant. The nuclear features are typical of papillary carcinoma and the cytoplasm is abundant and eosinophilic. In the columnar cell variant, the appearance has been likened to secretory endometrium.[15] The Hürthle cell variant of papillary carcinoma must be distinguished from the more common Hürthle variant of follicular carcinoma. Other variants are rare and include cribriform-morular, solid, oxyphil, Warthin's-like, trabecular, and tumor with nodular fasciitis-like stroma.

Differentiated Thyroid Cancer: Follicular Cancer (Chapter 5)

In the United States, follicular cancer accounts for 5%–10% of thyroid malignancies and the proportion increases in regions of iodine deficiency. The

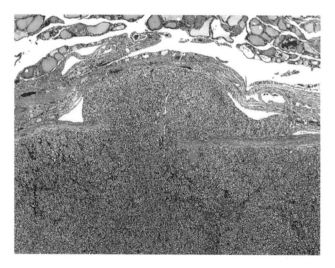

Figure 4.8. Capsular penetration is a hallmark of invasive well-differentiated follicular carcinoma (H&E ×250).

mean age is about a decade older than in papillary cancer and there is a 3:1 ratio of women to men. FNA of follicular cancer shows a repetitive micro-follicular pattern that is indistinguishable from follicular adenoma. The pathologic hallmarks for cancer are capsular invasion and vascular invasion.[16] Follicular cancer is further classified into either the minimally invasive or widely invasive types based on macroscopic and microscopic findings (Figure 4.8).

Variants of Well-Differentiated Follicular Cancer (Chapter 6)

Hürthle cell neoplasms can be adenomas or carcinomas and the pathologic differentiation can only be made by histopathologic examination. Hürthle cell carcinoma is usually a solitary mass and there can be central necrosis. Invasion into surrounding tissues can occur and is associated with a poorer outcome. Histologically, the cells are large polygonal with a granular eosinophilic cyto-plasm and prominent nucleoli.[17] Nuclear pleomorphism and mitotic activity including atypical forms can be present.

Poorly Differentiated Carcinoma: Insular Carcinoma (Chapter 6)

This cancer is uncommon in the United States. The lesions are large (>5 cm) and display invasive margins grossly. The histopathologic features include well-delineated nests or islands (insulae) surrounded by delicate fibro-vascular strands. At high power magnification, the neoplastic cells display small round nuclei, minimal pale cytoplasm, and are arranged in small clus-ters. The prognosis is poor.

Anaplastic Thyroid Cancer (Chapter 9)

FNA of anaplastic cancer shows a very cellular pattern with necrosis and the cells are usually pleomorphic and variable in size, shape, and appearance. These malignancies are usually very large with infiltration of surrounding tissues including muscles and trachea at the time of presentation. There are abundant regions of necrosis and hemorrhage. A variety of histologic patterns can be observed often with variation within the tumor itself (Figure 4.9). In some cases, a spindled or nonkeratinizing epidermoid pattern is present. There is usually no immunoreactivity for Tg or TTF-1, thus these cancers in a sense lack thyroidal differentiation. Treatment involves multimodality thera-pies but the prognosis is dismal.

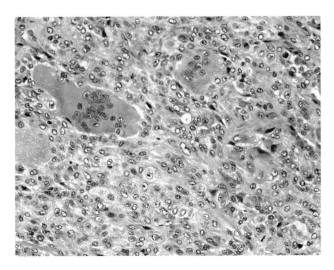

Figure 4.9. Anaplastic carcinoma containing multinucleated giant cells (H&E ×400).

Carcinoma of C Cell Origin: Medullary Thyroid Cancer (Chapter 10)

Approximately 25%–30% of patients with medullary cancer belong to families with familial medullary cancer or MEN 2A and 2B syndromes. Mutations in the *RET* protooncogene cause malignant transformation of the cells.[18,19] Cells that contain the mutation develop C cell hyperplasia and then micro-cancers and finally clinically apparent disease. FNA demonstrates a very cellular specimen and the cells are plasmacytoid, elongated or spindle-shaped in appearance. Amyloid deposits are found in about 50% of the FNA specimens and demonstrate apple-green birefringence under polarized light on Congo red stain. The most common site of medullary cancer is the lateral aspect at the junction of the upper one third and lower two third of the lobes. Sporadic cancers are usually solitary and can have a central fibrous scar and sharply circumscribed or infiltrative borders. The cells are arranged in lobules, trabeculae, nests, or sheets and are separated by amyloid deposits in about 80% of cases (Figure 4.10).

Hematolymphoid Neoplasms (Chapter 11)

Malignant lymphoma arising in the thyroid accounts for about 2%–5% of thyroid cancers and about 2.5% of lymphomas.[20] The patient is usually a

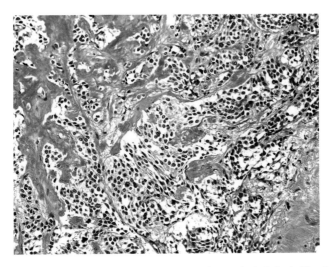

Figure 4.10. Medullary carcinoma demonstrating abundant amyloid admixed with cells with stippled chromatin (H&E ×300).

woman aged 60 years or older. There is a close association with pre-existing Hashimoto's thyroiditis with an estimated 80-fold increased risk of lymphoma.[21] Because diagnosis can be made by FNA with flow cytometry, there is less need for excisional biopsy. The cell of origin is the B lymphocyte and 10%–30% of the cancers are classified as MALTomas (mucosa-associated lymphoid tissue) or extranodal marginal zone B cell lymphoma of MALT.[22]

Hodgkin's lymphoma involving the thyroid is very uncommon. Diagnostic Reed-Sternberg cells and immunohistochemical support should be sought to establish the diagnosis.

Mesenchymal Tumors of the Thyroid

Angiosarcoma is the most important and common of the malignant mesenchymal tumors. A geographic predilection for the Alpine regions of Europe was reported.[23] Most patients are elderly and present with rapid enlargement of a preexisting thyroid mass. The tumors are large with abundant hemorrhage and necrosis (Figure 4.11).

Malignant teratoma is an extremely rare intrathyroidal cancer.[24]

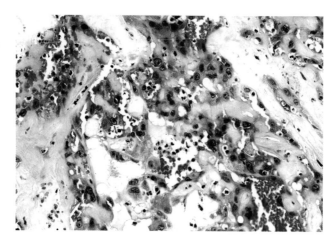

Figure 4.11. Angiosarcoma of the thyroid with irregular blood-filled vascular spaces lined by pleomorphic, hyperchromatic endothelial cells (H&E ×400).

Metastases to the Thyroid (Chapter 12)

Hematogenous spread to the thyroid is reported in a number of cancers including melanoma, carcinoma of the lung, breast, gastrointestinal tract, and renal cell carcinoma.[25–31]

Squamous Cell Carcinoma

Primary squamous cell carcinoma of the thyroid gland is rare. When a patient has a known cancer in a region close to or adjacent to the thyroid, a new mass in the thyroid can be the result of direct extension. Seventeen cases were collected at the Mayo clinic and 16 were squamous cell cancers of the larynx or esophagus.[32] The combination of FNA sampling and knowledge of the history should establish the correct diagnosis.

References

1. Nayar R, Frost AR. Thyroid aspiration cytology: a "cell pattern" approach to interpretation. Semin Diagn Pathol 2001;18(2):81–98.
2. Castro MR, Gharib H. Thyroid fine-needle aspiration biopsy: progress, practice, and pitfalls. Endocr Pract 2003;9(2):128–136.

3. Ranchod M. Thyroid gland. In: Ranchod M, ed. Intraoperative Consultations in Surgical Pathology. Philadelphia: Hanley & Belfus; 1996:389–403.

4. Rosai J. Immunohistochemical markers of thyroid tumors: significance and diagnostic applications. Tumori 2003;89(5):517–519.

5. Nikiforov Y. Recent developments in the molecular biology of the thyroid. In: Lloyd RV, ed. Endocrine Pathology: Differential Diagnosis and Molecular Advances. Totowa, NJ: Human Press; 2004:191–209.

6. Rosai J, Carangiu ML, DeLellis RA, eds. Tumors of the Thyroid Gland. Washington, DC: Armed Forces Institute of Pathology; 1992:161–182.

7. Hedinger C, Williams ED, Sobin LH. Histological typing of thyroid tumors. In: Hedinger CE, ed. International Histological Classification of Tumours. Vol 11. 2nd ed. Berlin: Springer-Verlag; 1988.

8. Williams E, Abrosimov A, Bogdanova T, et al. Two proposals regarding the terminology of thyroid tumors. Int J Surg Pathol 2000;8:181–183.

9. Brook I. Microbiology and management of acute suppurative thyroiditis in children. Int J Pediatr Otorhinolaryngol 2003;67(5):447–451.

10. Avram AM, Sturm CA, Michael CW, Sisson JC, Jaffe CA. Cryptococcal thyroiditis and hyperthyroidism. Thyroid 2004;14(6):471–474.

11. Kon YC, DeGroot LJ. Painful Hashimoto's thyroiditis as an indication for thyroidectomy: clinical characteristics and outcome in seven patients. J Clin Endocrinol Metab 2003;88(6):2667–2672.

12. Weetman AP. Autoimmune thyroid disease. Autoimmunity 2004;37(4):337–340.

13. Liu LH, Bakhos R, Wojcik EM. Concomitant papillary thyroid carcinoma and Hashimoto's thyroiditis. Semin Diagn Pathol 2001;18(2):99–103.

14. Egsgaard Nielsen V, Hecht P, Krogdahl AS, Andersen PB, Hegedus L. A rare case of orbital involvement in Riedel's thyroiditis. J Endocrinol Invest 2003;26(10): 1032–1036.

15. Rosai J, Kuhn E, Carcangiu ML. Pitfalls in thyroid tumour pathology. Histopathology 2006;49:107–120.

16. Li Volsi V. Surgical Pathology of the Thyroid. Philadelphia: WB Saunders; 1990:173.

17. Heppe H, Armin A, Calandra DB, Lawrence AM, Paloyan E. Hürthle cell tumors of the thyroid gland. Surgery 1985;98(6):1162–1165.

18. Eng C. RET proto-oncogene in the development of human cancer. J Clin Oncol 1999;17(1):380–393.

19. Santoro M, Melillo RM, Carlomagno F, et al. Molecular biology of the MEN2 gene. J Intern Med 1998;243(6):505–508.

20. Souhami L, Simpson WJ, Carruthers JS. Malignant lymphoma of the thyroid gland. Int J Radiat Oncol Biol Phys 1980;6(9):1143–1147.

21. Holm LE, Blomgren H, Lowhagen T. Cancer risks in patients with chronic lymphocytic thyroiditis. N Engl J Med 1985;312(10):601–604.

22. MacDermed D, Thurber L, George TI, Hoppe RT, Le QT. Extranodal nonorbital indolent lymphomas of the head and neck: relationship between tumor control and radiotherapy. Int J Radiat Oncol Biol Phys 2004;59(3):788–795.

23. Kim NR, Ko YH, Sung CO. A case of coexistent angiosarcoma and follicular carcinoma of the thyroid. J Korean Med Sci 2003;18(6):908–913.

24. Craver RD, Lipscomb JT, Suskind D, Velez MC. Malignant teratoma of the thyroid with primitive neuroepithelial and mesenchymal sarcomatous components. Ann Diagn Pathol 2001;5(5):285–292.

25. De Ridder M, Sermeus AB, Urbain D, Storme GA. Metastases to the thyroid gland: a report of six cases. Eur J Intern Med 2003;14(6):377–379.

26. Giuffrida D, Ferrau F, Pappalardo A, et al. Metastasis to the thyroid gland: a case report and review of the literature. J Endocrinol Invest 2003;26(6):560–563.

27. Haraguchi S, Hioki M, Yamashita K, Orii K, Matsumoto K, Shimizu K. Metastasis to the thyroid from lung adenocarcinoma mimicking thyroid carcinoma. Jpn J Thorac Cardiovasc Surg 2004;52(7):353–356.

28. Heffess CS, Wenig BM, Thompson LD. Metastatic renal cell carcinoma to the thyroid gland: a clinicopathologic study of 36 cases. Cancer 2002;95(9):1869–1878.

29. Kihara M, Yokomise H, Yamauchi A. Metastasis of renal cell carcinoma to the thyroid gland 19 years after nephrectomy: a case report. Auris Nasus Larynx 2004;31(1):95–100.

30. Lam KY, Lo CY. Metastatic tumors of the thyroid gland: a study of 79 cases in Chinese patients. Arch Pathol Lab Med 1998;122(1):37–41.

31. Nakhjavani MK, Gharib H, Goellner JR, van Heerden JA. Metastasis to the thyroid gland. A report of 43 cases. Cancer 1997;79(3):574–578.

32. Nakhjavani MM, Gharib MFH, Goellner MJ, Heerden MBCJA. Direct extension of malignant lesions to the thyroid gland from adjacent organs: report of 17 cases. Endocr Pract 1999;5(2):69–71.

5. Differentiated Thyroid Cancer

Introduction and Presentation

Papillary and follicular cancer cells retain the functions of trapping iodine and producing thyroglobulin (Tg). These cancers are grouped together as differentiated thyroid cancer. They are 3 times more common in women and the average age is 30–40 years. A new thyroid nodule or growth of an existing nodule is the usual presentation. Occasionally, a regional node containing metastatic cancer draws attention to the disease. A distant metastasis is a rare presentation. Fine needle aspiration of a new thyroid nodule or enlarged cervical node is recommended. Thyroid function is usually normal. Left untreated, the cancer will grow and cause pressure, difficulty breathing and swallowing, and metastasize to regional lymph nodes. A change in voice or hoarseness is a sign that the cancer has invaded the recurrent laryngeal nerve. There is increasing evidence of familial clusters of differentiated thyroid cancer; therefore, a new nodule in a first-degree relative who has thyroid cancer should be subjected to fine needle aspiration.

Natural History of Differentiated Thyroid Cancer

Most differentiated thyroid cancers grow slowly. The long-term outcome is excellent in patients who have been treated by surgery and thyroid hormone, or surgery, radioactive iodine (^{131}I), and thyroid hormone. The best prognosis is in patients younger than age 50 years. Women have a slightly better prognosis than men. Small (<2 cm) intrathyroidal cancers are associated with an excellent outcome. Invasion into surrounding tissues such as the trachea and distant metastases are poor prognostic factors. Metastasis to lymph nodes is associated with more recurrences but death from the cancer is not increased. An accurate prognosis can be predicted based on the age of the patient, the size of the cancer, and whether there are invasion and/or distant metastases.

Most authorities use the postoperative tumor/node/metastasis (pTNM) staging as shown in Table 5.1. A patient younger than 45 years with no distant metastasis is Stage I. The presence of a distant metastasis only increases this patient's stage to II. In contrast, a patient 45 years or older with a nodal metastasis is Stage III, as is a patient with a cancer larger than 4 cm. A patient with a distant metastasis is Stage IV.

Table 5.1. Thyroid cancer pTNM staging

Primary tumor	T0	No evidence of primary cancer
T1	T1	Tumor <2 cm
T2	Tumor >2–4 cm	
T3	Tumor >4 cm	
T4*	T4	Tumor of any size extending beyond the thyroid capsule
Regional nodes	N0	No regional lymph node metastasis
	N1	Regional lymph node metastasis
	N1a	Ipsilateral cervical nodes
	N1b	Bilateral midline or contralateral cervical or mediastinal nodal metastasis
Distant metastasis	M0	No distant metastasis
	M1	Distant metastasis
Younger than 45 years		
Stage I	Any T, any N, M0	
Stage II	Any T, any N, M1	
Stage III	Not applicable	
Stage IV	Not applicable	
45 years or older		
Stage I	T1, N0, M0	
Stage II	T2, N0, M0	
Stage III	T3, N0, M0, or any T, N1, M0	
Stage IV	Any T, any N, M1	

There are several systems that use criteria such as age, size of the primary cancer, and presence of distant metastases to provide a numeric score that defines outcome. The mnemonic MACIS, abbreviated from Metastasis, Age, Completeness of resection, Invasion, and Size, provides a quantitation of the mortality risk.[1] The formula is age multiplied by 0.08 (or 3.1 if aged <40 years), plus size of cancer in centimeters multiplied by 0.3, +1 for incomplete excision, +1 for local invasion, and +3 points for a distant metastasis. Several other prognostic indices use similar input factors. "Staging" patients allows prognostication and makes it possible to compare treatments among patients with similar extent of disease. pTNM is used internationally and is recommended. MACIS provides an excellent alternative and one that patients understand easily.

Fundamentals of Treatment

The principle of treatment is to remove all cancerous cells. This requires thyroidectomy. Some surgeons recommend a total thyroidectomy over a lesser procedure. The reasons for this disparity in opinion are discussed along with the pros and cons of the operations. Small cancers are often confined to the thyroid and therefore are removed by thyroidectomy. Metastases to regional lymph nodes can be treated by operation or radioiodine ^{131}I or both. Metastases to distant sites, usually lung and or bone, less commonly brain, soft tissues, and liver must be treated on an individual basis but ^{131}I is used most often. After thyroidectomy, the patient requires thyroid hormone for life. It is possible to reduce growth of differentiated thyroid cancer cells and their production of Tg by prescribing a dose of levothyroxine, which reduces thyrotropin (TSH).

Surgery

The key to management of differentiated thyroid cancer is a skilled thyroid surgeon. There is general but not unanimous consensus that a total thyroidectomy is the operation of choice. Some surgeons argue for a lesser procedure especially in low-risk patients. Patients who are Stage I or who have a MACIS score of <6 are very unlikely to die from thyroid cancer. These patients are usually young and a complication of the operation such as permanent hypoparathyroidism can be very troublesome. A permanent paralysis of the recurrent laryngeal nerve can interfere with jobs that require lecturing, speaking in public, or singing. Several authorities recommend lobectomy in these situations.[2,3]

There are fewer recurrences in patients who have had a more complete thyroidectomy.[4] Fifty-four percent of patients undergoing completion of thyroidectomy had cancer in the contralateral lobe.[5] However, a clinical recurrence in the residual lobe is less common and in one series was only 4%.[6] Treatment with ^{131}I is easier when there is less residual thyroid and there are fewer complications such as radiation thyroiditis. In addition, the diagnostic whole-body scan and posttreatment scan are more likely to show functioning metastases on the first postoperative evaluation. Measurement of Tg for follow-up of patients is more reliable when most of the thyroid has been removed. Total (or near total) thyroidectomy is the preferred procedure but has to be balanced against the risks of the operation. When a lesser operation is undertaken and the primary cancer is <1.5 cm and fully excised the patient should have an excellent prognosis. When the cancer is larger, locally invasive, or there are nodal metastases, a total thyroidectomy is advised. When only a lobe was removed, completion of thyroidectomy and ^{131}I ablation is advised.

The operation should be conducted by a surgeon who has been trained in the procedure and who has had experience with many thyroidectomies. The surgeon should also have a very low complication rate. The patient should meet with the surgeon and take a written list of questions concerning the procedure, risks, recovery time in hospital, time for recuperation, whether the surgeon identifies the recurrent and superior laryngeal nerves or uses nerve monitoring, and the involvement by trainees, etc. An accompanying relative or close friend is helpful. In complicated operations such a "redo" procedure when the first operation did not remove sufficient gland, the surgeon should be the one who has experience in this situation where the complication rate is recognized to be higher. The incision is usually about 1–1.5 finger breadths (2–3 cm) above the sternal notch. The incision is still called a Kocher incision after Emil Theodor Kocher who reduced the operative mortality from 14% in 1884 to 0.18% in 1898. He received the Nobel Prize in physiology and medicine in 1909. The use of mini-incisions and video-assisted thyroidectomy has been conducted with no increase in complications. It remains to be proven whether this is appropriate for patients with thyroid cancer when total thyroidectomy and selective lymph node dissection are necessary.

Death, hemorrhage, hypoparathyroidism, recurrent and superior laryngeal nerve paralysis, and difficulty swallowing are the main complications. Some patients are unhappy with the scar and a keloid is very unsightly and difficult to correct. Complications are more frequent after total thyroidectomy and total thyroidectomy plus neck dissection.[7] They are also more common during reoperation and in the hands of surgeons conducting small numbers of thyroidectomies.[8] The main immediate risks of thyroidectomy are the life-threatening ones. Postoperative bleeding and hematoma formation are of great concern because unless treated expeditiously can cause compression of the trachea and death. Postoperative bleeding occurred in 0.7%–1.59% of 21,680 thyroidectomies. In an older report, the mortality in patients older than 70 years was 0.66% compared with 0.02% for those younger than 50 years. Nevertheless, thyroidectomy can be completed successfully in the elderly as one report in 12 patients older than 80 years confirms.[9] None of 14,934 patients in a multicenter study died but a permanent complication occurred in 7.1%[10]; 1.3% had recurrent laryngeal nerve injuries and 3.3% hypocalcemia. In an analysis of 5583 patients from the United States (US), 9.8% of the low-risk patients (T1N0M0) had a complication (79% of these were hypocalcemia).[11] This is important because these patients have an excellent prognosis and they are usually young and have to live with the complication for the rest of their life.

Hypocalcemia from permanent hypoparathyroidism requires large doses of calcium (2–3 g daily) plus 0.25–0.5 μg 1:25 dihydroxycholecalciferol. During surgery where all parathyroids appear to have been compromised, one gland can be autotransplanted into a pocket in the sternocleidomastoid or the forearm. There is a role for local anesthesia in older patients, those with cardiovascular disease, and pregnant women. One group uses local anesthesia as their standard and have experience with more than 600 patients.[12]

In summary, total or near total thyroidectomy is the operation of choice and the quality of the operation is central to the management. The published incidences of permanent hypothyroidism and recurrent laryngeal nerve paralysis are higher than 1% for each (the generally quoted acceptable percentage). An experienced surgeon capable of removing the thyroid with a low complication rate is a huge advantage.

Radioactive Iodine

Radioactive iodine treatment is usually preceded by a diagnostic whole-body scan using a radionuclide of iodine and ^{123}I is being used more often as the diagnostic radionuclide. For therapy, ^{131}I, which has been used for more than 60 years, is used exclusively.[13] Follicular cells transport iodine against an electrochemical gradient from serum to cell. The molecular structure of the trapping mechanism is located in the laterobasal segment of the cell. It transports one atom of iodide and two atoms of sodium and hence is known as the sodium iodide symporter (NIS).[14,15] TSH controls the gene that encodes NIS as well as its function. Other tissues including salivary gland, breast, stomach, thymus, kidney, and choroid plexus express NIS. These organs can be seen on whole-body scans using radionuclides of iodine. NIS in thyroid cancer cells is present in reduced amounts or it is not targeted to the correct site, thus cancers trap less iodine than normal follicular cells.[16]

The treating physician should meet with the patient to outline the protocol and to ensure that the patient understands this is a protracted procedure. TSH should be increased and this has usually been achieved by withdrawal of thyroid hormone resulting in symptomatic hypothyroidism. Advice is given about a low iodine diet. Potential side effects of radioactive iodine are described. A discussion of radiation safety issues and precautions is included.

Diagnostic Scanning

A diagnostic scan determines how much residual thyroid has been left after thyroidectomy and defines the presence of functioning metastases (Figure 5.1). It also determines whether treatment with ^{131}I is appropriate and in follow-up whether treatment with ^{131}I has been successful, or not. It also ensures the proposed high dose of therapeutic ^{131}I does not irradiate a physiologic site such as the breasts. An increased TSH is necessary for trapping of iodine. This is achieved after total or near total thyroidectomy by waiting 4 weeks without thyroid hormone replacement. Most authorities recommend values >30 mU/L but I hope to have the value >50 mU/L. When the patient has been started on thyroid hormone postoperatively there are two approaches. Levothyroxine is stopped for 4 weeks or it is replaced by triiodothyronine for 4 weeks. Then the triiodothyronine is stopped for 12–14 days and equivalent TSH values are found.[17] Brans et al.[18] confirm that the diagnosis of cancer, the worry about treatment with internal radiation, the need for isolation, and hypothyroidism,

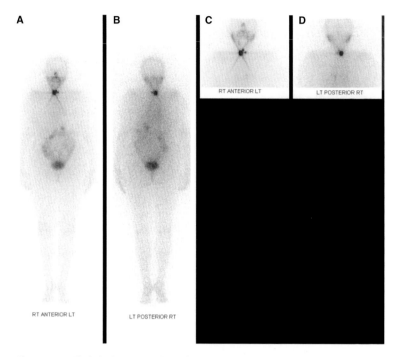

Figure 5.1. Whole-body anterior **(A)** and posterior **(B)** scintiscans and spot views of the anterior **(C)** and posterior **(D)** neck and chest. The images were made 24 hours after 2 mCi (74 MBq) ^{123}I. There is uptake in the thyroid bed and a small focus in the left neck likely attributable to metastasis in a lymph node. There is physiologic uptake in salivary glands, stomach, intestines, and bladder.

all lead to depression and anxiety. This is worsened by the hypothyroid condition. Whole-body scan and measurement of stimulated Tg in the patient for follow-up can be obtained after withdrawal of thyroid hormone, or injection of recombinant human TSH (rhTSH).

Recombinant Human Thyrotropin

Ladenson et al.[19] reported on the use of rhTSH in a phase III trial in 127 patients. The patients had a whole-body diagnostic scan after two intramuscular injections of 0.9 mg of rhTSH on consecutive days. A scan was obtained

48 hours after 2–4 mCi (74–148 MBq) [131]I. The patients then had a diagnostic scan after withdrawal of thyroid hormone. Eighty-three percent of the paired scans were concordant. Of the 21 discordant pairs, 18 were positive on the withdrawal scan but negative after injection of rhTSH, i.e., the standard preparation was superior. A second phase III trial was conducted using 4 mCi (148 MBq) [131]I and measurement of stimulated Tg in 229 patients.[20] There was concordance in 89%. One hundred percent with metastatic disease were identified by rhTSH scan and Tg. Side effects from rhTSH were mild but about 10% of the patients reported headache or nausea after the injection of rhTSH. Patients do not develop antibodies after repeated injections of rhTSH.[21] The Food and Drug Administration (FDA) approved the use of rhTSH for diagnostic scanning in December 1998. I have conducted more than 260 diagnostic scans after rhTSH stimulation. Preliminary results have been published.[22,23] Thirteen percent had a transient headache and 21% had mild nausea. The mean TSH 24 hours after the second injection was >120 mU/L. Ninety percent diagnostic whole-body studies were negative and Tg values ≤ 5 ng/mL, which I accept as not meriting additional tests or treatment. When the stimulated value was ≥ 10 ng/mL and the scan was negative, additional testing was undertaken to try to identify the site of Tg production.

TSH stimulus can cause growth of lesions resulting in pain, respiratory problems, and central nervous system complications such as hemiparesis. Therefore, precautions should be taken in patients who have cancer in critical areas such as the spine. This applies to withdrawal of thyroid hormone and injection of rhTSH.

Some authorities advocate measurement of a stimulated Tg alone as sufficient and omit the diagnostic scan.[24] One review makes the point that approach is acceptable after a negative follow-up scan and Tg have been achieved.[25] My preference is to obtain at least one follow-up scan and stimulated Tg because there are reports of undetectable Tg in patients with known residual cancer.[26] When both are negative, stimulated Tg values could be used after that. In patients with no residual disease, repeated tests with rhTSH are reliable and consistent.

Low Iodine Diet

The goal of diagnostic imaging and therapy is to have thyroid cells trap as much radioiodine as possible. The average daily intake of iodine in the US is 200–500 µg. When dietary iodine intake is high, the diagnostic and therapeutic tracers of radioactive iodine are diluted by the nonradioactive [127]I. Most authorities recommend a low iodine diet for 2 weeks before testing and treatment. One source of a large dose of iodine is radiographic contrast and a delay of 6–8 weeks is advised after this has been injected. Amiodarone has a high concentration of iodine and a very long half-life and testing and treatment have to be delayed for up to a year provided the medication can be stopped.

Which Radioactive Tracer?

[131]I was used for diagnostic whole-body imaging for decades. However, there were concerns that the diagnostic scan on occasion did not provide as detailed an analysis as the posttherapy scan. Several authorities did not find a significant difference.[27,28] There was added concern that diagnostic doses of ^{131}I could damage the trapping ability of thyroid cells so that therapeutic ^{131}I would be concentrated in lower amounts and not be so effective in killing the cancer cells. This is called "stunning." For this reason, it is reasonable to restrict the dose of ^{131}I to 1–3 mCi (37–111 MBq) [131]I. Because of the drawbacks of ^{131}I, ^{123}I, a pure gamma (γ) emitter with a half-life of 13 hours, is now used more frequently. The 159 keV energy of the γ of ^{123}I is suited to high-resolution imaging with a γ camera and some consider it the ideal radionuclide in this situation.[29] Several investigators have shown its value and high sensitivity for whole-body scanning.[30–33] Published test doses of ^{123}I vary from <37 MBq (<1.0 mCi) to 185 MBq (5.0 mCi); I use 4 mCi (148 MBq) and images are obtained after 24 hours. [131]I is administered orally as a capsule or liquid and whole-body scan is conducted after 48–72 hours. There is some evidence that the sensitivity of ^{131}I scan is greatest at 72 hours after administration of [131]I.

Interpretation of the Whole-Body Scan

Anterior and posterior whole-body scans and anterior and posterior spots of the neck and chest are obtained with the patient lying supine. Multiple spot views are acceptable but more difficult to interpret. It is important that a low-energy collimator is used for ^{123}I and a high-energy one for ^{131}I, or the scans can be impossible to interpret (Figure 5.2). A quantitative measurement of the percentage uptake over the thyroid bed and functioning lesions is obtained using a probe. Radioiodine is trapped wherever there is NIS and normal thyroid traps most avidly. Functioning metastases in regional lymph nodes and distant sites are identified provided there is not excessive residual normal thyroid (Figures 5.3A and B and 5.4). Other organs seen on the scan include the salivary glands and stomach. The bladder is usually seen on scans made over the first 2–3 days. Scans made later often show uptake in the colon and rectum. Active breast tissue can be imaged, and testing and treatment should be deferred for some months after lactation.[34] The liver can be imaged on scans made several days after treatment (Figure 5.5).

Figure 5.2. Two sets of anterior and posterior scintiscans made after the patient had been treated with ¹³¹I. A low-energy collimator was used instead of high-energy (the γ emissions from ¹³¹I of 365 keV are too high for regular collimator) and the images are uninterpretable. The study was not conducted at Stanford.

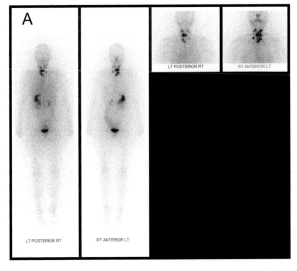

Figure 5.3. A Whole-body scan and spot views made 24 hours after 4 mCi (148 MBq) ¹²³I. There is uptake of ¹²³I in residual thyroid and functioning nodal metastases.

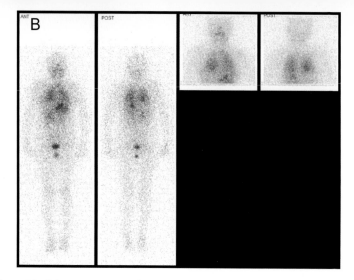

Figure 5.3. B Posttreatment scan demonstrating pulmonary metastases in whole-body and spot scintiscans. The patient had been treated 7 days earlier with 150 mCi (5.5 GBq) ^{131}I.

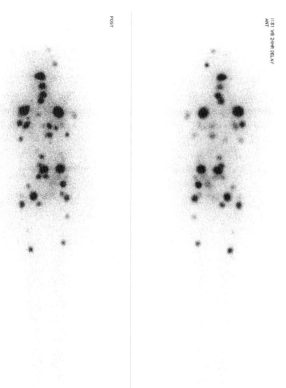

Figure 5.4. Whole-body scan demonstrating widespread skeletal metastases. This was obtained 7 days after treatment with ^{131}I.

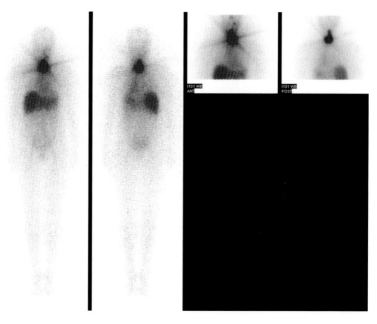

Figure 5.5. Anterior and posterior whole-body scans and spot views of the neck and chest made 7 days after treatment with ^{131}I. There is a large residuum of thyroid and this produced radioiodinated thyroid hormones that are metabolized in the liver.

False-Positive Findings

There are several comprehensive reviews of reports of benign or nonthyroid cancer disorders that have caused difficulty on interpretation, also shown in Table 5.2.[35,36] Excreted radioactivity in saliva, urine, and occasionally feces are potential causes of false-positive results (Figures 5.6 and 5.7). Several nonthyroidal cancers can occasionally trap iodine. There are several reports of uptake in the thymus, mostly in young patients on the posttherapy scan (Figure 5.8).[37]

Table 5.2. List of false-positive findings on whole-body scan based on previous tabulations by the author[35,36]

Site	Disorder
Head	Meningioma
	Wig, hair, scalp
	Artificial eye
	Dacryocystitis
	Subdural hematoma
Nose	Sinusitis, "hot nose"
Salivary glands	Physiologic, sialoadenitis, Warthin's tumor
Mouth	Saliva
	Periodontal disease, oral disease
	Chewing tobacco
	Lingual thyroid
Neck outside thyroid bed	Tracheostomy
	Thyroglossal duct
	Carotid ectasia
Thorax and lungs	Cancer
	Inflammatory lung disease, bronchiectasis
	Pleural effusion
	Bronchogenic cyst
Cardiac	Pericardial effusion
	Struma cordis
	Pleuropericardial cyst
Thymus	Physiologic
Breast	Lactating, or recent pregnancy
	Breast cyst
Esophagus	Barrett's esophagus
	Esophageal stricture
	Zenker's diverticulum
	Hiatal hernia
Liver	Diffuse uptake: physiologic uptake on late "posttreatment" scans
	Focal uptake: probable functioning metastases
Biliary tract	Gallbladder
	Dilated intrahepatic duct
Stomach	Physiologic
	Gastric carcinoma
Colon	Physiologic
	Meckel's diverticulum
	Colonic graft
Urinary tract	Physiologic on early scans, renal cyst, polycystic kidneys, ectopic kidney
Reproductive system	Ovary, ovarian cystadenoma, struma ovarii
	Endometriosis
Contamination	Contaminated handkerchief
Perspiration	Perspiration in axillae, perspiration under a watch

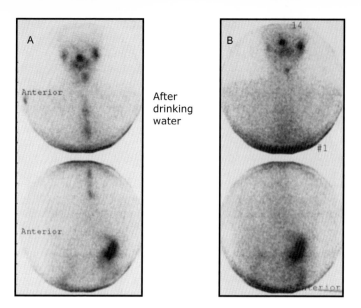

Figure 5.6. **A** Linear concentration of radioiodine in the central thorax. **B** This activity disappeared after the patient drank water, confirming that it was in the esophagus.

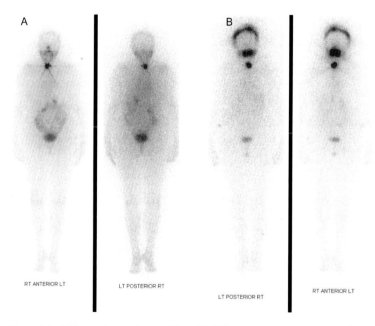

Figure 5.7. **A** Diagnostic scan after 4 mCi (148 MBq) ^{123}I. **B** A posttreatment scan 1 week after administration of ^{131}I. The major difference is diffuse uptake over the top of the head in the posttherapy scan. This was attributed to radioactive saliva used to keep the hair look fashionable.

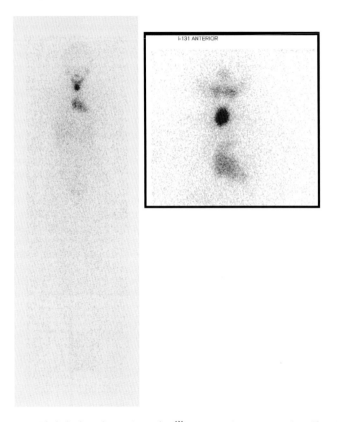

Figure 5.8. Whole-body and spot views after ^{131}I treatment in a young patient. There is a remnant of uptake in the thyroid bed and uptake in the central chest, which is typical of thymus.

Thyroglobulin

Tg measurement is valuable in patients who have had surgical and ^{131}I treatment. The level of Tg is dependent on the level of TSH and the size and site of residual thyroid, particularly thyroid cancer. Approximately 25%–30% of patients with papillary thyroid cancer have anti-Tg.[38] Endogenous antithyroglobulin antibodies compete with antibodies used for the assay. There is a dilemma as to the diagnostic value of the Tg measurement when anti-Tg is present. In addition, different Tg assays can give different results in the same sample. Radioimmunoassays are one-step procedures; immunoradiometric assays (IRMA) and chemoluminescent assays are two-step assays. In most patients, there is a close relationship between the measurement of Tg and whole-body scan findings; in other words, both are positive or both are negative. A measurable (increased) Tg with a negative scan is a management dilemma and is discussed under controversies. An increase in Tg usually represents an increase in the mass of thyroid cancer provided TSH is constant and the same assay used. Very large quantities of Tg swamp the capacity of the anti-Tg antibody that captures Tg in the first step of IRMA and produces a lower value, which is called the hook effect.

Treatment with Thyroid Hormone

All patients who have had thyroidectomy need thyroid hormone. Well-differentiated thyroid cancer responds to TSH, thus TSH levels should not be persistently high. However, high doses of thyroid hormone can have adverse effects on the cardiovascular system, the skeleton, and on the brain. In thyrotoxicosis, there is increased bone resorption, reduced trabecular bone, and osteoid surface, and an increase in the resorptive surface. Bone density measurements are reduced. Several investigators confirm a reduction of bone density in the radius, hip, spine, or calcaneus.[39] However, dual energy X-ray absorptiometry measurements in 49 patients with treated thyroid cancer who had higher T_4 and lower TSH levels were similar to normal, age-matched controls.[40] Greenspan and Greenspan[41] in a metaanalysis of published research, concluded that suppression of TSH can reduce bone density in pre- and post-menopausal women. Older women with prolonged suppression of TSH are at most risk of developing reduced bone density and have increase in hip and vertebral fracture.

Cardiac manifestations of thyrotoxicosis include tachycardia, palpitations, ectopic beats, atrial fibrillation, increased pulse pressure, left ventricular hypertrophy, and high output cardiac failure. Sawin et al.[42] found a threefold increase in atrial fibrillation in patients older than 60 years. Anxiety, nervousness, difficulty sleeping, irritability, and anger can result from too much thyroid hormone.

In patients with newly diagnosed and treated low-risk cancer, it is reasonable to have the TSH in the range close to the lower end of normal, for example, 0.1–0.6 mU/L. After a period of follow-up showing a negative scan and low values of Tg, the TSH could be titrated to the range of 0.3–1.0 mU/L. There would be no increased risks from the medication or the disease. In contrast, in patients with high-risk cancer, or persistent disease despite appropriate treatments, there is a role for prescribing more thyroid hormone to keep the TSH lower. The dose is usually just less 1 μg per pound body weight. L-Thyroxine is the preferred medication and there are six FDA-approved preparations that are not interchangeable. Klein and Danzi[43] have reviewed the therapeutic efficacy of L-thyroxine preparations and make the point that when a substitution is made there is considerable risk that the TSH level can change and can put the patient at risk for subclinical thyroid dysfunction. Thyroid hormone should be taken several hours apart from calcium and iron. All pregnant women who have no thyroid reserve need to increase their intake of L-thyroxine during pregnancy.[44,45] They should also take supplementary iron and vitamins at a different time.

Treatment with Radioiodine [131]I

The goal of therapy is to deliver enough damage to the diseased cells to kill them and at the same time deliver as little toxic effects to nonthyroidal tissues as possible so that complications are absent or mild. [131]I treatment can deliver remarkably high doses of radiation to the desired sites at little expense to the remainder of the body. [131]I was first administered by Seidlin. The patient had thyrotoxicosis as a result of functional metastases 19 years after thyroidectomy.[46] The patient improved considerably and functioned well for several years after ^{131}I therapy.

[131]I is administered to remove residual thyroid left after near total or subtotal thyroidectomy, so-called remnant ablation. However, the first treatment can be designed to deal with regional or distant metastases provided the surgeon has removed the primary cancer and all or nearly all normal thyroid. Some endocrinologists treat postoperatively by ordering a "fixed" routine dose without a diagnostic scan. This ignores how much tissue is present and percentage uptake of radioiodine and whether there are functioning metastases. The dose could be too small for some patients or inappropriately large for others. [131]I is also used to treat thyroid metastases.

A brief discussion of radiation physics is introduced. The absorbed radiation to thyroid tissue is dependent on the volume of residual thyroid, the quantity of ^{131}I administered, the percentage uptake of the administered dose in the thyroid tissues, and its effective half-life at that site. The most common approach to calculate the absorbed radiation is called the MIRD method (Medical Internal Radiation Dose Committee of the Society of Nuclear Medicine). The word dose has two meanings. First, dose applies to the quantity of radiation administered. This is in units of becquerel, usually mega or giga becquerel in the SI system, or curies, usually millicurie in the standard system. One becquerel produces one emission per second and 1 mCi gives off 3.7×10^7 emissions per second. One hundred millicurie is equivalent to 3.7 GBq and 1 GBq is equivalent to 27 mCi. The second use of dose refers to the quantity of radiation deposited in or absorbed by tissues. The SI unit for absorbed dose is the gray and that is equal to 1 joule of energy deposited in 1 kg of tissue. The standard unit is the rad (radiation absorbed dose) which is equal to 100 ergs deposited in 100 g. One joule is equal to 10^7 ergs, therefore 1 Gy equals 100 rad, alternatively 1 rad is equal to 1 cGy or 10 mGy. It is useful to know that 1 μCi (37 Bq) [131]I delivers 0.433 rad (0.433 cGy) to 1 g of tissue in 1 hour. This number can be used to calculate how much radiation is delivered when the administered dose, the size of the lesion, the percentage uptake, and half-life of the radioiodine are known. The physical half-life $T_{1/2p}$ of ^{131}I is 8.04 days or 193 hours. The biologic half-life $T_{1/2B}$ is the time to the turn over half the iodine by the body. The effective half-life $T_{1/2E}$ is derived from the formula:

$$\frac{1}{T_{1/2E}} = \frac{1}{T_{1/2P}} + \frac{1}{T_{1/2B}}$$

The effective half-life of ^{131}I in functioning thyroid including metastases along with the number of microcuries per gram of tissue determines the success of therapy.

Empiric Therapy for "Ablation of Remnants"

The goal should be to administer the lowest dose that will eradicate 100% of cells in 100% of patients.[47] One dose does not fit all. A dose of 29.9 mCi (1.1 GBq) was popular because in many countries and in the US until recently that was the maximum administered dose that was allowed for out-patient therapy (NRCP report no. 37). This dose works provided there is a small volume of tissue with a low percentage of uptake.[48] A randomized study of eight different administered doses ranging from 15 mCi (555 MBq) to 50 mCi (2.2 GBq) showed there was a statistically significant benefit from doses of 25 mCi (925 MBq) or greater.[49] Low doses should not be administered to a patient with locally invasive cancer or metastases to lymph nodes or distant sites. Significant multifocal disease would weigh against low-dose treatment.

Beierwaltes et al.[50] reported an 87% success rate in 233 patients with thyroid tissue confined to the thyroid bed using a dose of 100 mCi (3.7 GBq). Hoyes et al.[51] conducted a retrospective analysis of 60 patients treated with 95 mCi (3.5 GBq) ^{131}I. The average uptake was 18.4% and they successfully ablated 54 of 60 (90%) defined as <1.0% on follow-up scan after a delay of 3 months.

Some recommend fractionated therapy, i.e., three doses of 30 mCi at intervals of about a week, instead of a single dose of approximately 100 mCi. Problems include whether there is a need for second and third administrations because the first fraction might be all that is required. Second, there must be concern that the first treatment could cause "stunning" so that subsequent doses would not be trapped (see controversies later in this chapter). Third, there would be the need for radiation safety requirements for outpatients for several weeks rather than days. Finally, the patient would be hypothyroid considerably longer. This is not recommended.

In summary, when it appears that the patient would be successfully ablated by one small dose based on a low uptake and little residual thyroid, proceed that way. In other situations, prescribe a dose that will have a high likelihood of working, e.g., 100–150 mCi (3.5–5.5 GBq). Then deal with the logistics as dictated by country or state.

Treatment of Metastases: Empiric Therapy

Functioning lymph node metastases would usually be treated with 100–175 mCi (3.7–6.5 GBq). Pulmonary metastases are usually treated with 150–200 mCi (5.5–7.4 GBq) and skeletal lesions with 200 mCi (7.4 GBq). These empiric doses do not take into consideration the mass of cancer, the percentage uptake, or the $T_{1/2EFF}$. The outcome in patients with nodal and micronodular pulmonary metastases is good when patients are treated this way. Massin et al.[52] treated 58 patients with pulmonary metastases that constituted 7% of their total group. They administered 100–200 mCi (3.7–7.4 GBq) for lung lesions and the 8-year survival for those with micronodular disease was 77%. Schlumberger et al.[53] treat with fixed doses of 100 mCi (3.7 GBq) and repeat the treatment after 6 months. When the cancer could be ablated using ^{131}I, 89% survived for 15 years. [131]I seldom causes radiation fibrosis and this is discussed below under complications of radioiodine treatment. The outcome in patients with macronodular pulmonary disease is guarded.

Bone metastases are often lytic and when they are in a weight-bearing site, a radiation oncologist and orthopedist should be consulted for advice. [131]I in a dose of 200 mCi (7.4 GBq) is administered and repeated after 1 year when there is continued uptake of radioiodine in lesions. The 10-year survival from the time of metastases is 10%–20%.

Dosimetry to Deliver a Specific Absorbed Radiation Dose to the Cancer

The calculations required to derive that 1 μCi in 1 g for 1 hour deposits 0.433 rad are beyond the scope of this book but can be found in reference.[54] The volume of tissue being treated must be known plus the percentage retention of radioiodine and its effective half-life. Then it is possible to determine what dose of ^{131}I should be administered to deliver, for example, 30,000 rad.[55]

Dosimetry Using Diagnostic [124]I

[124]I, which is a positron emitter with a 4-day half-life, has been used for dosimetry. Three-dimensional, high-resolution images can be generated.[56] Approximately 2–4 mCi (74–148 MBq)[124]I is administered and imaged at 4, 20, 44 hours and after 4–6 days. Accurate measurement of the absorbed dose is possible not only for individual lesions but for different regions within a lesion.

Dosimetry to Ensure Marrow and Lung and Total-Body Radiation Are Not Excessive

Hematologic complications occur when the blood receives 200 rad (2 Gy) or more.[57] Retention of 120 mCi (4.4 GBq) at 48 hours delivers a cumulative dose of 200 rad (2 Gy) to the blood. Severe pulmonary complications occur when the lungs retain 80 mCi or more (≥ 2.96 GBq) at 48 hours after treatment. Sisson[58] has presented a simplified method of dosimetry. The method is to measure whole-body retention of a diagnostic dose of ^{131}I at 2 hours and use this as the 100% baseline. A repeat measurement is made after 48 hours and the retention used to ensure the administered dose could not result in retention of 120 mCi (4.4 GBq). A diagnostic scan demonstrating where the activity is located could be used along with the percentage retention. One of the sources of total-body radiation is from ^{131}I-labeled thyroid hormone. Sisson also recommends measuring FT_4 based on the principle that the higher that value the more likely there will be high levels of radioiodinated thyroid hormones and excessive blood, marrow, and whole-body irradiation.[59] The administered dose is empirically reduced by 10%–20% when the FT_4 is between 0.25 and 1 ng/dL, by 20%–40% for an FT_4 between 1.0 and 1.8 ng/dL, and by 40%–60% for a value >1.8 ng/mL. Prevention of retention of 80 mCi (2.94 MBq) in the lungs is achieved by calculating the percentage of whole-body radioactivity from a diagnostic dose that is retained in a region of interest over the thorax. Dosimetry is not required in most patients but when there is a desire to deliver a specific absorbed dose to a lesion, it is obviously necessary. When there are widespread functioning metastases including multiple skeletal or pulmonary lesions, it is important to determine that the marrow and lungs are not exposed to an excess absorbed dose.

Treatment After Stimulation with Recombinant Human Thyrotropin

rhTSH has not been approved for treatment by the FDA but has been in the European Union. The use of rhTSH for treatment is exciting but there are still some facts that need to be resolved. The efficacy of rhTSH stimulation versus hypothyroidism in the ablation of thyroid remnants is the same.[60,61] Nine patients with Stage I or II disease were studied first when euthyroid after 2 doses (4 patients) or 3 doses (5 patients) of rhTSH then when hypothyroid.[62] The blood clearance was faster in the euthyroid state but the percentage uptake in lesions was greater as was the residence time. rhTSH had a 5.7 times advantage over the hypothyroid condition, therefore therapy with ^{131}I would produce a higher radiation to the lesion but the blood and whole-body radiation would be less. The use of rhTSH for both remnant ablation and treatment of functioning metastases is expanding. More data will be needed to define its exact role versus withdrawal of thyroid hormone including what administered dose of ^{131}I is optimal.

Regulations for Release of Radioactive Patients

The regulations for release of patients who have been treated with ^{131}I differ from country to country and practitioners must know and adhere to those rules that apply. The US regulations are discussed here. The current regulations of the US Nuclear Regulatory Commission revised Title 10 of the code of Federal Regulations (10 CFR 35.75) allow release of patients with a retained dose of ≤ 33 mCi (≤ 1.22 GBq) and emitted radiation of ≤ 7 mrem/h at 1 m.[63] When it can be documented that no adult person could be exposed to 500 mrem (5 mSv), the patient can be released. For this, it is then necessary to develop a formula using the distance in meters and the inverse square rule, the occupancy time, the actual emitted radiation at 1 m at the time of treatment to determine whether outpatient treatment is appropriate. The exposures of 65 family members of 30 patients who were treated as outpatients were measured.[64] The mean dose to relatives was 0.24 mSv (24 mrem with a range of 10–109 mrem), which was well below the limit (5.0 mSv).

Because of concern that terrorists might set off a dirty bomb or release radioactivity, airports now have radiation detectors. Patients generally would not be flying soon after ^{131}I therapy but if there is an emergent need, a document should be provided that they have been treated with details of dose and date. Apparently, all alarms that have gone off have been attributed to medical rather than terrorist sources of radiation.[65]

Side Effects and Complications

The preparation, including hypothyroidism, low iodine diet, radiation precautions, and long-term follow-up, is weighty and time-consuming. In addition, side effects have been reported in 77% of patients in one study (Table 5.3).[66] TSH can stimulate growth of cancer in an enclosed space. There is a need to consider surgery, external radiation, or cyber knife before proceeding to treat a mass lesion within a fixed space with [131]I. Nausea is common after large doses of ^{131}I and the patient can be given prophylactic medication. Experience with one, such as ondansetron (Zofran), is advised.

Radiation thyroiditis produces pain over the thyroid bed that radiates to the jaw and ear. The symptom can start as early as 1 day after treatment but is most common between 2–5 days. The pain is worsened by swallowing and talking. The skin over the thyroid is red and the area is extremely sensitive to touch. This complication is usually found when the surgeon has left a substantial volume of thyroid. Transient thyrotoxicosis caused by release of thyroid hormone might follow. Antiinflammatory medications given in adequate doses are helpful but if the symptoms persist after 24 hours a short course of prednisone has a dramatic effect.

The salivary symptoms are not common in patients receiving <3.7 GBq (100 mCi). A transient change or loss of taste occurs days to weeks after [131]I

Table 5.3. Side effects and complications of ^{131}I treatment

Early side effects	Late side effects
Growth of cancer by TSH stimulation	Permanent hypothyroidism
Thyroiditis	Xerostomia
Transient thyrotoxicosis	Dry eyes, also tearing
Sialadenitis	Reduced sperm counts
Loss or change of taste	Reduced fertility
Stomach pain	Increased risk of congenital abnormalities
Nausea	Increased incidence of cancer (leukemia, breast, and bladder)
Vomiting	Early menopause
Neck edema	Radiation pneumonitis and fibrosis
Recurrent laryngeal nerve paralysis	Reduced parathyroid function
	Anaplastic transformation of cancer

treatment. Sialadenitis was found in 33% (67 of 203 patients).[66] Methods to reduce sialadenitis include sucking lemon candy and lemon drops to encourage salivary flow and to ensure the patient is well hydrated. There is debate regarding when the prophylactic lemon should be started, but most advise at the time of ^{131}I administration. The use of amifostine seems to have helped reduce the incidence and severity of sialadenitis.[67] The glands become swollen and tender and the onset can be within 24 hours of treatment. On rare occasions, the glands become symptomatic weeks or months after ^{131}I therapy and a proportion of patients end up with a dry mouth. An increase in salivary gland tumors has been identified in one report.[68]

Lacrimal dysfunction has occurred in 92% of patients. Chronic conjunctivitis occurred in 27% of treated patients.[66] There are reports of blockage of the nasolacrimal duct after [131]I.[69]

When ^{131}I is administered, there is a theoretic risk of leukemia and this was described early after the introduction of ^{131}I therapy for thyroid cancer.[70,71] Pochin[72] found three patients with leukemia among those he had treated in the 1950s. This number was statistically greater than 0.25 cases expected based on the size of the treated population. These three patients had all received more than 1050 mCi (38.9 GBq). The patients were treated with substantial doses at shorter intervals than is current practice. Chronic myeloid leukemia has been identified in several patients. When standard doses are used at intervals of more than 6 months, the risk is low.

Iodine can be concentrated by NIS in breast cells and there are several reports of breast uptake on whole-body scans using radioiodine.[34,73,74] There is increasing concern about a relationship of breast cancer occurring after treatment of thyroid cancer. The implication is that ^{131}I causes the breast cancer. Alternatively, thyroid cancer is a disease of young women and breast cancer a disease of older women. Therefore, it would not be unexpected for one cancer to follow the other. Also, the women might have a genetic predisposition for cancer in general. One report showed a 1.5 relative risk for breast cancer after a diagnosis of thyroid cancer and also a relative risk of 1.5 for thyroid cancer after a diagnosis of breast cancer.[75] An increased risk of breast cancer (relative risk 1.18) was identified in 252 women after they had thyroid cancer.[76] However, when women were premenopausal at the time of diagnosis and treatment of thyroid cancer, the relative risk was 1.49 ($P < .001$). There was a significant excess of these cancers in women younger than 59 years out of 2365 women treated for thyroid cancer in three French Cancer Centers.[77] There should be a degree of caution when treating young women who have low risk thyroid cancer with [131]I.

A statistically significant increase in bladder cancer has been described.[78] In 2113 pregnancies evaluated in women treated for thyroid cancer, there was a slight increase in miscarriage after surgery and radioiodine therapy compared with before any intervention.[79] This was more likely related to thyroid dysfunction than to [131]I. There was no difference in the "incidences of stillbirth, preterm birth, low birth weight, congenital malformation and death during the first year of life before or after ^{131}I therapy." Transient problems with menses were found in 17% of young women treated with ^{131}I but no permanent effect on the ovaries and 276 of the women bore 427 children.[80] Pacini and colleagues[81] demonstrated a higher follicle stimulating hormone in 103 men who had been treated on average 15 months before. The dose to the gonads was 6.4 cGy (6.4 rad) after 3 GBq (80 mCi), 14.1 cGy (14.1 rad) from 5.5 MBq (150 mCi), and 21.2 cGy (21.2 rad) from a cumulative dose of 9.2 GBq (250 mCi).[82] When it might be necessary to prescribe repeated large therapeutic doses, sperm could be banked. Women who received ^{131}I had an earlier menopause than women given suppressive doses of L-thyroxine to treat goiter.[83]

Radiation pneumonitis and fibrosis after ^{131}I has been described.[84] The complication seems rare but the absence of new data and the adverse outcomes in historic references are difficult to explain. The consensus is that a retained dose of 80 mCi or more ($\geq$ 2.96 GBq) [131]I in the lungs should be avoided.

In summary, ^{131}I is well tolerated compared with systemic chemotherapy and external radiation therapy. Nevertheless, there are early and late complications, some of which are troublesome such as permanent dry mouth and some clinically serious such as second cancers. The expected benefits of treatment have to be weighed against the risks for the individual patient. In the case of a small cancer ($\leq$ 2 cm) that has been fully excised in a young patient, it is hard to decide that the balance favors therapy.

Posttherapy Scintiscan

It is now routine to image the distribution of ^{131}I several days after its administration. This is judged to be a sensitive investigation and several authors report that more lesions are identified in comparison to pretreatment diagnostic scan (Figure 5.9). I find this is seldom the case either for diagnostic

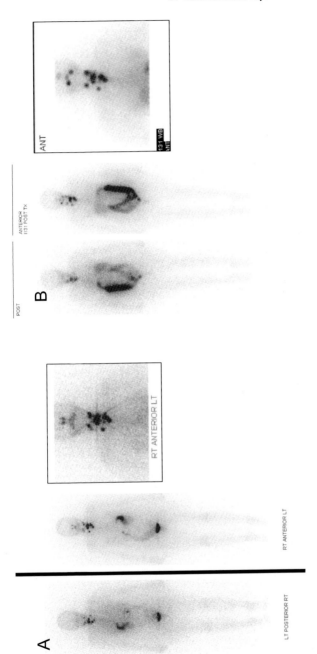

Figure 5.9. **A, B** Whole-body anterior and posterior as well as spot views of the neck and chest. **A** After 4 mCi (148 MBq) ^{123}I. **B** Posttherapy scan 1 week after ^{131}I. There is no difference in distribution in the neck. The posttreatment scan shows bowel activity caused by radioiodinated hormones being excreted through the bile into the gastrointestinal tract.

[131]I or ^{123}I imaging. This is confirmed by other investigators.[28,85] Nevertheless, it is valuable to demonstrate that the treatment localized as intended. This can also be used as a time to remeasure the emitted radiation and determine if the radiation safety instructions can be withdrawn.

Follow-Up After Treatment of Cancer

After treatment by surgery and ^{131}I it is important for the patient to be followed long-term. Recurrences can occur and although most do so in the first 5 years, a minority can occur over decades. There is no consensus about a single investigation, or group of tests, but all are of the opinion that follow-up for a long time is required. My approach is to check thyroid function and Tg 8 weeks after therapy. The TSH would be adjusted depending on the severity of the cancer. In most patients, the goal would be a value between 0.1–0.6 mU/L. Tg would be compared with the pretreatment value and used for comparison with subsequent measurements. An undetectable value is very reassuring. Six months after therapy, a follow-up visit would include physical examination of the neck, measurement of thyroid function, and Tg. After 1 year, a whole-body scan with measurement of a stimulated Tg is obtained along with physical examination. An ultrasound of the neck can be included at this time and some authorities might include that at the 6-month visit. There are differences of opinion about the value of the diagnostic scan at this time. In the low-risk patient, some omit the scan and measure a stimulated Tg. As discussed previously, I prefer both. It is helpful and reassuring for the patient to see the before-treatment and follow-up scans. In those with high-risk cancer, all would accept that scan and Tg should be measured. The lack of consensus here is whether the patient should be hypothyroid, or euthyroid and given injections of rhTSH. The decision is best based on whether it is likely the patient would need a second treatment with [131]I. Therefore, when the Tg remains elevated and residual tissue is present, thyroid hormone would be withdrawn. When Tg values are low or undetectable, the scan could be conducted using rhTSH. Some authorities have a policy to repeat scans annually for 5 years but that approach has gradually been altered in favor of less imaging. Some physicians plan for two scans. When the first follow-up scan is negative and the Tg is <2 ng/mL, I arrange visits at 6-month intervals for physical examination, thyroid function, and Tg measurement and occasional ultrasound. At 5 years, a second follow-up scan is obtained using rhTSH stimulation and Tg is measured at that time. After that, annual visits are arranged until the 10-year anniversary and then depending on patient level of concern the visits are organized at 1- to 2-year intervals. When the patient needs a second treatment with ^{131}I or has a late recurrence, the type of testing and frequency of clinic visits increases until a stable situation is reached.

In the patient who is treated by operation and no [131]I (see below), visits are arranged at intervals of 6 months to palpate the neck and measure TSH and

Tg. Periodic ultrasounds are usually obtained annually for 2–3 years and then biannually.

External Radiation as an Alternative to [131]I

Although there is a role for external radiation in a patient with anaplastic cancer, skeletal metastases of differentiated thyroid cancer that do not trap ^{131}I, and invasive medullary cancer, it has no role in the routine management of patients with Stage I and II or low MACIS or AGES (age, grade of tumor, extent of tumor, tumor size) scores. External radiation damages the cells without killing all of them. The cancer then fails to trap ^{131}I but can also become more aggressive in behavior. Carr et al.[86] in 1958 called this a "common error in the treatment of carcinoma of the thyroid."

Controversies

There are many controversial aspects on the management of differentiated thyroid cancer. This is difficult to understand because the prognosis is excellent and most patients survive a normal lifespan and live normal, productive lives. It is true that some patients have a relapse but these can usually be treated successfully. Why is there so much controversy? One reason is that there are no controlled trials. A second reason is related to the excellent prognosis that results in physicians believing that they alone are responsible for that outcome. The controversy about how much thyroid should be removed by operation has been covered and is not repeated. Controversy about the dose or preparation of thyroid hormone has also been covered. Here the topics are related to radioactive iodine therapy.

Is [131]I Necessary?

Earlier in the chapter, the review of the results of several investigators seemed to demonstrate improved outcome in patients treated with [131]I. Those with metastases whose cancers trapped iodine and were treated with ^{131}I lived longer. The therapy can be shown to work by removing functioning tissue and scintiscans after therapy demonstrate that thyroid cells in the thyroid bed or in sites of metastases can no longer be imaged and have been successfully ablated. Serum Tg values decrease after treatment and in many patients become undetectable. It is comforting, even exciting, for patient and physician to see the improved results on scan and serum tests. However, does the treatment reduce the rate of recurrence or improve survival? Where is the objective data from a controlled trial in matched patients randomly selected for ^{131}I therapy or placebo managed by a defined protocol? Reliance has to be placed on decision models, metaanalysis, or retrospective evaluations. In one computer model of a patient with localized cancer, there was an improvement in life expectancy of 4–8 months and the reduction in recurrence was deemed to outweigh the risk of leukemia.[87]

Models cannot and do not take all factors into consideration. In the study under discussion, leukemia was the only complication of ^{131}I treatment that was considered. These investigators also determined that it would be necessary to enroll 4000 patients and follow them for 25 years to demonstrate a 10% improvement in mortality. Sawka et al.[88] presented a metaanalysis of whether remnant ablation is effective. They confirm that they did not identify one randomized, controlled study. They identified 23 articles that met stringent inclusion criteria. Although the data from different reports were inconsistent, when the data were pooled there was a reduction in recurrence (relative risk 0.31) and a slight reduction in distant metastases. The authors point out that distant metastases are rare and in their analysis only occurred in 4% of those who did not receive [131]I. The article concludes, "In the meantime, the decision for RAI (radioactive iodine) ablation must be individualized based on the risk profile of the patient, as well as the patient and physician preference, while balancing the risks and benefits."

The investigators did not address complications from the treatment. A permanently dry mouth is very unpleasant and can lead to dental caries and although not life-threatening, cannot be condoned in patients who would not benefit from [131]I. The same applies to a small increase in cancer. Editorials accompanying the original article come down on the side of favoring the radioiodine treatment. Mazzaferri[89] argues that ablation allows accurate measurement of a stimulated Tg and a negative posttherapy ^{131}I scan. The destruction of microscopic foci of cancer has theoretic and probably real value. He identifies the reduction in mortality from thyroid cancer in women over recent years; however, this is in part attributable to earlier diagnosis. Haugen[90] entitles his contribution "Patients with Differentiated Thyroid Carcinoma Benefit from Radioiodine Remnant Ablation" and concludes that older patients and those with large cancers and lymph node metastases have a better outcome when treated with [131]I. He also confirms prior analysis that "the benefit of radioiodine in younger patients with smaller tumors is less clear, and the potential risks of therapy need to be thoroughly considered."

Several retrospective analyses show an advantage from [131]I.[5] Mazzaferri and Jhiang[4] conducted a very detailed retrospective analysis of 1322 patients with differentiated thyroid cancer who at onset did not have distant metastases. Twenty-three percent received treatment with radioiodine. The investigators found that older age, large cancer size, and local invasion increased the risk of recurrence significantly. The relative risk of recurrence was 0.4 (95% confidence intervals 0.2–0.9, $P < .05$) in those treated with [131]I. The cancer-specific mortality was 8% after 30 years. In these and all other reports concerning ^{131}I, it is difficult to know what were the clinical features or personal biases that led to treatment of some patients but not others. The outcome was improved by ^{131}I in 303 patients treated in 14 US and Canadian centers.[91]

Eighty-five percent of those with papillary cancer received this and there was a reduction in cancer-specific mortality and progression of disease. The benefit was not statistically significant when patients with tall cell variant (to be discussed below) were excluded. The authors conclude that "this study supports improvement in overall and cancer-specific mortality among patients with papillary and follicular thyroid cancer after postoperative iodine-131 therapy." A cancer registry including 2282 patients from 76 hospitals in Illinois confirms an improvement in survival after ^{131}I treatment.[92]

In contrast, Hay et al.[93] have reported on the outcome in 2444 patients with papillary cancer treated at the Mayo clinic. No difference in cancer-related mortality or recurrence of cancer in 1917 patients with MACIS <6.0 was identified in those treated with ^{131}I versus those who were not treated. The authors do recommend ^{131}I for high-risk patients with MACIS scores $\geq$ 6.0 who are at greater risk of recurrence or death. In my experience, only 5.6% of patients treated by thyroidectomy and no ^{131}I were subsequently treated by operation, ^{131}I, or both.[94] Contrary to conventional advice, Tg measurement was valuable in this group and was low or undetectable and remained constant.

Not all patients with differentiated thyroid cancer need treatment with [131]I. Young patients with early disease have such a good prognosis that it would not be possible to demonstrate a benefit. Evidence shows no reduction in recurrence or mortality in patients with MACIS scores <6.0 who are treated with [131]I. Older patients, those with locally invasive disease, regional and or distant metastases have less recurrences and mortality when treated.

Stunning?

Stunning is the term given when a diagnostic dose of radioiodine (^{131}I) causes enough radiation to thyroid cells that the therapeutic dose of ^{131}I is not able to be concentrated by those cells and the effect of therapy is compromised.[95] Park et al.[96] demonstrated that as the diagnostic dose increased, there was an increasing percentage of patients whose posttherapy scan showed reduced uptake. Other reports demonstrating stunning have been published.[97,98] Data opposed to the concept include the fact that ^{131}I has been used successfully for decades, there were no data describing this effect over decades, plus several studies show no such effect.[27,99] An in vitro experiment demonstrated that as the absorbed dose of radiation increased from 1 to 30 Gy (100–3000 rad) the transport of iodine from the basal membrane to the apex decreased. However, a recent unpublished report from the same group shows this is time related and trapping is increased for 2–3 days after radiation and then decreases. This almost certainly explains the disparate reports. Those who do not find stunning treat immediately after the diagnostic scan; those who find stunning treat later. An alternative explanation is that iodine is taken up and released from different regions of thyroid tissue at different rates (Figure 5.10).

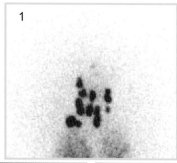

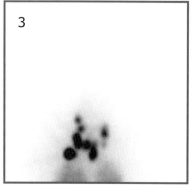
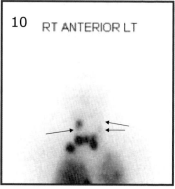

Figure 5.10. Spot views of the neck 1, 3, and 10 days after ^{123}I and treatment with [131]I. With the passage of time, the number of abnormal nodes imaged becomes less. Therefore, images at 10 days might be interpreted as showing stunning, but the correct interpretation is differential rates of wash-out of ^{131}I from nodes.

Thyroglobulin-Positive, ^{131}I-Negative Patients

Not all patients who have negative scans have undetectable Tg values. This indicates there are thyroid cells, most likely malignant, somewhere. It should be kept in mind that Tg is not incorporated in any of the staging or prognostic indices.[100] Technical factors should be reviewed including the TSH value, energy settings of the camera, and possible exposure to iodine. Then there are three approaches: one is to wait, two to treat with a high dose of ^{131}I, and three to use alternative imaging tests. Most patients with differentiated thyroid cancer have an excellent prognosis, the mortality is low, and there is probably no risk of waiting provided the patients are kept under observation and Tg is measured periodically.

Data in favor of treatment with a large dose of ^{131}I include identifying uptake on a posttherapy scan and finding a decrease in Tg.[101,102] There are no data to show prognosis is improved and some that it might be worsened by this approach.[103,104] My experience in selected patients is that none was improved, none had a significant decrease in Tg, and most required additional tests to identify the source of Tg. High-dose ^{131}I should not be advised when there is obvious clinical disease. That should be treated by surgery or external beam therapy depending on its site. High-dose ^{131}I might have a role when there is no evidence of bulky disease in a patient who has a clear understanding of the controversy who also recognizes that the Tg value will rarely become undetectable. Figure 5.11A shows a diagnostic whole-body scan that is almost negative (very faint lung uptake). Figure 5.11B shows significant lung uptake after treatment with [131]I. This would be taken to favor empiric therapy; however, the Tg value did not change, which must be considered as an argument against this approach.

The third approach is to try to identify the source of Tg production by an alternative imaging test or tests. Ultrasound is excellent but is dependent on the size of nodes. However, criteria such as roundness, hypoechogenicity, loss of the fatty hilum, and increased vascularity increase the sensitivity of the test. Historically, thallium (^{201}Tl), ^{99m}Tc-sestamibi, ^{99m}Tc-tetrafosmin, and ^{111}In-

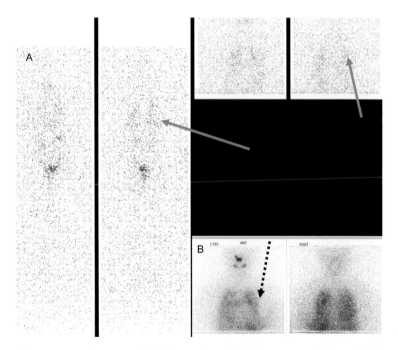

Figure 5.11. **A** A diagnostic whole-body scan that is almost negative (very faint lung uptake) and is not an absolute Tg positive, iodine negative. **B** Significant lung uptake after treatment with [131]I. However, the Tg value did not decrease.

octreotide have been used but these have been replaced by positron emission tomography (PET) and PET/computed tomography (CT) using [18]FDG (fluoro-deoxyglucose). Combined PET/CT provides functional images of FDG plus attenuation correction and also provides anatomic images that can be read side by side with the PET images. Combined PET/CT can explain that FDG uptake is in muscles or brown fat rather than nodes, and false positives can be reduced. Patients with high levels of Tg are more likely to have positive PET scans, and lesions smaller than 5 mm are often too small to be identified. Intense uptake of FDG is a poor prognostic indicator and these lesions are more likely to be resistant to ^{131}I treatment.[105] My experience with PET alone is in more than 102 patients and with PET/CT in 90 studies. The latter had a sensitivity of 87% and specificity of 80%. There might be an advantage from a high TSH. Figure 5.12 is an example of PET/CT in a patient with negative radioiodine scintiscan.

Our approach is that, after a lesion is identified by PET/CT, it is biopsied usually under ultrasound guidance. At surgery, intraoperative ultrasound pinpoints the lesion, which is excised, and an immediate intraoperative ultrasound at that time demonstrates that the lesion is no longer there.[106] Pre-operatively, 11 of 13 had increased Tg values with a mean of 10.5 ng/mL

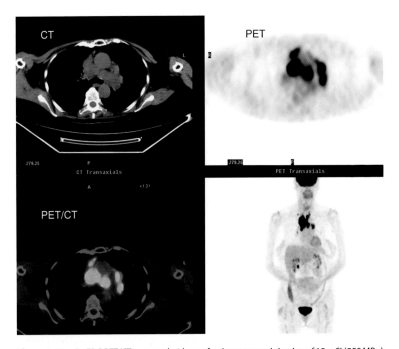

Figure 5.12. An FDG PET/CT scan made 1 hour after intravenous injection of 15 mCi (555 MBq) [18]FDG. The patient had a negative iodine scan and high Tg. There is intense uptake of FDG in mediastinal and hilar nodes. Treatment with ^{131}I would be futile and potentially harmful.

whereas TSH was low. Tg decreased in all patients to a mean of 0.84 ng/mL and in seven it became undetectable. Therefore, we would prefer this approach to treating Tg-positive, iodine-negative patients when the lesions are accessible.

Additional Methods of Treatment

External Radiation

When sites of thyroid cancer do not trap iodine and are in regions that are not suited to operation, they can be treated by external radiation.

Embolization of Cancer

Bulky symptomatic lesions, in particular those in the skeleton, can be reduced in size by embolization of their arterial supply using particles such as polyvinyl alcohol, sponges, or microcoils. Investigators interested in the procedure have administered therapeutic ^{131}I and after a short delay shrunk the lesion by arterial embolization.[107]

Methods to Induce Redifferentiation of the Cancer

Retinoic Acid

Retinoic acid increases mRNA for NIS in cultured thyroid cancer cells and increases trapping of radioiodine.[108] In patients, the dose is 1.5 mg/kg daily for at least 5 weeks. One report in 50 patients demonstrated that Tg values decreased or stabilized in 20 patients (40%).[109] Other investigators find the response to be disappointing and conclude, "An indiscriminate use of isotretinoin in all patients with otherwise untreatable thyroid cancer cannot be recommended."[110]

Lithium

Lithium inhibits the release of iodine and thyroid hormone from thyroid. This could increase the residency or $T_{1/2B}$ of the radioiodine. The data are mixed. Schraube et al.[111] reported that neither the uptake nor retention of ^{131}I was altered. A positive report described an increase in $T_{1/2E}$ of 50% and suggests this could be a useful adjunct.[112] When I have prescribed lithium, the uptake was still low and there seemed to be little benefit. Six hundred milligrams is administered followed by 300 mg three times a day with the aim of having a serum lithium between 0.6–1.2 mEq/L.

References

1. Hay I, Bergstralh EJ, Goellner JR, Ebersold JR, Grant CS. Predicting outcome in thyroid carcinoma: development of a reliable prognostic scoring system in a cohort of 1779 patients surgically treated at one institute during 1940 through 1989. Surgery 1993;114:1050–1058.

2. Shaha AR, Shah JP, Loree TR. Low-risk differentiated thyroid cancer: the need for selective treatment. Ann Surg Oncol 1997;4(4):328–333.

3. Shaha AR. Thyroid cancer: extent of thyroidectomy. Cancer Control 2000;7(3): 240–245.

4. Mazzaferri E, Jhiang SM. Long-term impact of initial surgical and medical therapy on papillary and follicular thyroid cancer. Am J Med 1994;97:418–428.

5. Mazzaferri E. Radioiodine and other treatment and outcomes. In: Braverman LE, Utiger RD, eds. Werner and Ingbar's The Thyroid. A Fundamental and Clinical Text. 8th ed. Philadelphia: Lippincott Williams & Wilkins; 2000:904–929.

6. Cady B. Presidential address: beyond risk groups—a new look at differentiated thyroid cancer. Surgery 1998;124(6):947–957.

7. Mazzaferri EL, Young RL, Oertel JE, et al. Papillary thyroid carcinoma: the impact of therapy on 576 patients. Medicine 1977;56:171–196.

8. Shaha A, Jaffe BM. Completion thyroidectomy: a critical appraisal. Surgery 1992;112:1148–1152.

9. Miccoli P, Iacconi P, Cecchini GM, et al. Thyroid surgery in patients aged over 80 years. Acta Chir Belg 1994;94(4):222–223.

10. Rosato L, Avenia N, Bernante P, et al. Complications of thyroid surgery: analysis of a multicentric study on 14,934 patients operated on in Italy over 5 years. World J Surg 2004;28(3):271–276.

11. Hundahl SA, Cady B, Cunningham MP, et al. Initial results from a prospective cohort study of 5583 cases of thyroid carcinoma treated in the United States during 1996. U.S. and German Thyroid Cancer Study Group. An American College of Surgeons Commission on Cancer Patient Care Evaluation study. Cancer 2000; 89(1):202–217.

12. Williams M, Lo Gerfo P. Thyroidectomy using local anesthesia in critically ill patients with amiodarone-induced thyrotoxicosis: a review and description of the technique. Thyroid 2002;12(6):523–525.

13. Seidlin S, Marinelli LD, Oshry E. Radioactive iodine therapy: effect on functioning metastases of adenocarcinoma of the thyroid. JAMA 1946;132:838–847.

14. Dai G, Levy O, Carrasco N. Cloning and characterization of the thyroid iodide transporter. Nature 1996;379:458–460.

15. Smanik PA, Liu Q, Furminger TL, et al. Cloning of the human sodium iodide symporter. Biochem Biophys Res Commun 1996;226(2):339–345.

16. Wapnir IL, van de Rijn M, Nowels K, et al. Immunohistochemical profile of the sodium/iodide symporter in thyroid, breast, and other carcinomas using high

density tissue microarrays and conventional sections. J Clin Endocrinol Metab 2003;88(4):1880–1888.

17. Goldman J, Line BR, Aamodt RL, et al. Influence of triiodothyronine withdrawal time on 131I uptake postthyroidectomy for thyroid cancer. J Clin Endocrinol Metab 1980;50:734–739.

18. Brans B, van den Eynde F, Audenaert K, et al. Depression and anxiety during isolation and radionuclide therapy. Nucl Med Commun 2003;24(8):881–886.

19. Ladenson P, Braverman LE, Mazzaferri EL, et al. Comparison of administration of recombinant human thyrotropin with withdrawal of thyroid hormone for radioactive iodine scanning in patients with thyroid carcinoma. N Engl J Med 1997; 337:888–896.

20. Haugen BR, Pacini F, Reiners C, et al. A comparison of recombinant human thyrotropin and thyroid hormone withdrawal for the detection of thyroid remnant or cancer. J Clin Endocrinol Metab 1999;84(11):3877–3885.

21. Paterakis T, Ebels H, Mallick UK, et al. Lack of antigenicity of recombinant human thyrotropin after multiple injections in patients with differentiated thyroid cancer. Thyroid 2000;10(7):623.

22. Durski JM, Weigel RJ, McDougall IR. Recombinant human thyrotropin (rhTSH) in the management of differentiated thyroid cancer. Nucl Med Commun 2000;21(6): 521–528.

23. McDougall I, Weigel RJ. Recombinant human thyrotropin in the management of thyroid cancer. Curr Opin Oncol 2001;13:39–43.

24. Mazzaferri EL, Massoll N. Management of papillary and follicular (differentiated) thyroid cancer: new paradigms using recombinant human thyrotropin. Endocr Relat Cancer 2002;9(4):227–247.

25. Robbins RJ, Robbins AK. Clinical review 156: recombinant human thyrotropin and thyroid cancer management. J Clin Endocrinol Metab 2003;88(5):1933–1938.

26. Westbury C, Vini L, Fisher C, Harmer C. Recurrent differentiated thyroid cancer without elevation of serum thyroglobulin. Thyroid 2000;10(2):171–176.

27. McDougall IR. 74MBq radioiodine 131I does not prevent uptake of therapeutic doses of 131I (i.e. it does not cause stunning) in differentiated thyroid cancer. Nucl Med Commun 1997;18:505–512.

28. Fatourechi V, Hay ID, Mullan BP, et al. Are posttherapy radioiodine scans informative and do they influence subsequent therapy of patients with differentiated thyroid cancer? Thyroid 2000;10(7):573–577.

29. Park HM. 123I: almost a designer radioiodine for thyroid scanning. J Nucl Med 2002;43(1):77–78.

30. Yaakob W, Gordon L, Spicer KM, Nitke SJ. The usefulness of iodine-123 whole-body scans in evaluating thyroid carcinoma and metastases. J Nucl Med Technol 1999;27(4):279–281.

31. Gulzar Z, Jana S, Young I, et al. Neck and whole-body scanning with 5-mCi dose of (123)I as diagnostic tracer in patients with well-differentiated thyroid cancer. Endocr Pract 2001;7(4):244–249.

32. Fenwick JD, Mallick UK, Perros P. 123I imaging in the follow-up of differentiated thyroid cancer. Clin Oncol (R Coll Radiol) 2001;13(4):314.

33. Cohen JB, Kalinyak JE, McDougall IR. Clinical implications of the differences between diagnostic 123I and post-therapy 131I scans. Nucl Med Commun 2004; 25(2):129–134.

34. Perros P, Mallick UK, Fenwick JD. Radioiodine uptake in normal female breasts and liver of a patient with differentiated thyroid cancer imaged by whole body scanning. Thyroid 2003;13(5):511.

35. McDougall IR. Whole-body scintigraphy with radioiodine-131. A comprehensive list of false positives with some examples. Clin Nucl Med 1995;20:869–875.

36. Carlisle M, Lu C, McDougall IR. The interpretation of 131I scans in the evaluation of thyroid cancer, with an emphasis on false positive findings. Nucl Med Commun 2003;24:715–735.

37. Davidson J, McDougall IR. How frequently is the thymus seen on whole-body iodine-131 diagnostic and post-treatment scans? Eur J Nucl Med 2000;27(4): 425–430.

38. Spencer CA, Takeuchi M, Kazarosyan M, et al. Serum thyroglobulin autoantibodies: prevalence, influence on serum thyroglobulin measurement, and prognostic significance in patients with differentiated thyroid carcinoma. J Clin Endocrinol Metab 1998;83(4):1121–1127.

39. Ross D. Hyperthyroidism, thyroid hormone therapy and bone. Thyroid 1994;4: 319–326.

40. Franklyn J, Betteridge J, Dykin J, et al. Long-term thyroxine treatment and bone mineral density. Lancet 1992;340:9–13.

41. Greenspan SL, Greenspan FS. The effect of thyroid hormone on skeletal integrity. Ann Intern Med 1999;130(9):750–758.

42. Sawin CT, Geller A, Wolf PA, et al. Low serum thyrotropin concentrations as a risk factor for atrial fibrillation in older persons. N Engl J Med 1994;331(19): 1249–1252.

43. Klein I, Danzi S. Evaluation of the therapeutic efficacy of different levothyroxine preparations in the treatment of human thyroid disease. Thyroid 2003;13: 1127–1132.

44. Mandel SJ. Hypothyroidism and chronic autoimmune thyroiditis in the pregnant state: maternal aspects. Best Pract Res Clin Endocrinol Metab 2004;18(2): 213–224.

45. McDougall IR, Maclin N. Hypothyroid women need more thyroxine when pregnant. J Fam Pract 1995;41(3):238–240.

46. Siegel E. The beginnings of radioiodine therapy of metastatic thyroid carcinoma: a memoir of Samuel M. Seidlin, M.D. (1895–1955) and his celebrated patient. Cancer Biother Radiopharm 1999;14(2):71–79.

47. Cooper DS, Doherty GM, Haugen BR, et al. Management guidelines for patients with thyroid nodules and differentiated thyroid cancer. Thyroid 2006;16(2): 109–142.

48. van Wyngaarden M, McDougall IR. What is the role of 1100 MBq (<30 mCi) radio-iodine 131I in the treatment of patients with differentiated thyroid cancer? Nucl Med Commun 1996;17(3):199–207.

49. Bal CS, Kumar A, Pant GS. Radioiodine dose for remnant ablation in differentiated thyroid carcinoma: a randomized clinical trial in 509 patients. J Clin Endocrinol Metab 2004;89(4):1666–1673.

50. Beierwaltes WH, Rabbani R, Dmuchowski C, Lloyd RV, Eyre P, Mallette S. An analysis of "ablation of thyroid remnants" with I-131 in 511 patients from 1947–1984: experience at University of Michigan. J Nucl Med 1984;25(12): 1287–1293.

51. Hoyes KP, Owens SE, Millns MM, Allan E. Differentiated thyroid cancer: radioiodine following lobectomy—a clinical feasibility study. Nucl Med Commun 2004;25(3):245–251.

52. Massin JP, Savoie JC, Garnier H, Guiraudon G, Leger FA, Bacourt F. Pulmonary metastases in differentiated thyroid carcinoma. Study of 58 cases with implications for the primary tumor treatment. Cancer 1984;53(4):982–992.

53. Schlumberger M, Challeton C, de Vathaire F, et al. Radioactive iodine treatment and external radiotherapy for lung and bone metastases from thyroid carcinoma. J Nucl Med 1996;37:598–605.

54. McDougall I. Management of Thyroid Cancer and Related Nodular Disease. London: Springer-Verlag; 2006:Chapter 5.

55. Maxon HR. Quantitative radioiodine therapy in the treatment of differentiated thyroid cancer. Q J Nucl Med 1999;43(4):313–323.

56. Sgouros G, Kolbert KS, Sheikh A, et al. Patient-specific dosimetry for 131I thyroid cancer therapy using 124I PET and 3-dimensional–internal dosimetry (3D-ID) software. J Nucl Med 2004;45(8):1366–1372.

57. Benua RS, Cicale NR, Sonenberg M, Rawson RW. The relation of radioiodine dosimetry to results and complications in the treatment of metastatic thyroid cancer. Am J Roentgenol Radium Ther Nucl Med 1962;87:171–182.

58. Sisson JC, Shulkin BL, Lawson S. Increasing efficacy and safety of treatments of patients with well-differentiated thyroid carcinoma by measuring body retentions of 131I. J Nucl Med 2003;44(6):898–903.

59. Sisson JC, Carey JE. Thyroid carcinoma with high levels of function: treatment with (131)I. J Nucl Med 2001;42(6):975–983.

60. Robbins RJ, Tuttle RM, Sonenberg M, et al. Radioiodine ablation of thyroid remnants after preparation with recombinant human thyrotropin. Thyroid 2001; 11(9):865–869.

61. Pacini F, Ladenson PW, Schlumberger M, et al. Radioiodine ablation of thyroid remnants after preparation with recombinant human thyrotropin in differentiated thyroid carcinoma: results of an international, randomized, controlled study. J Clin Endocrinol Metab 2006;91(3):926–932.

62. Luster M, Sherman SI, Skarulis MC, et al. Comparison of radiobiokinetics following the administration of recombinant human thyroid stimulating hormone and after

thyroid hormone withdrawal in thyroid carcinoma. Eur J Nucl Med Mol Imaging 2003;30:1371–1377.

63. Tuttle WK 3rd, Brown PH. Applying Nuclear Regulatory Commission guidelines to the release of patients treated with sodium iodine-131. J Nucl Med Technol 2000; 28(4):275–279.

64. Grigsby PW, Siegel BA, Baker S, Eichling JO. Radiation exposure from outpatient radioactive iodine (131I) therapy for thyroid carcinoma. JAMA 2000;283(17): 2272–2274.

65. Gangopadhyay KK, Sundram F, De P. Triggering radiation alarms after radioiodine treatment. BMJ 2006;333(7562):293–294.

66. Alexander C, Bader JB, Schaefer A, Fincke C, Kirsch C-M. Intermediate and long-term side effects of high-dose radioiodine therapy for thyroid carcinoma. J Nucl Med 1998;39:1551–1554.

67. Bohuslavizki KH, Klutmann S, Jenicke L, et al. Salivary gland protection by S-2-(3-aminopropylamino)-ethylphosphorothioic acid (amifostine) in high-dose radioiodine treatment: results obtained in a rabbit animal model and in a double-blind multi-arm trial. Cancer Biother Radiopharm 1999;14(5):337–347.

68. Dottorini ME, Lomuscio G, Mazzucchelli L, Vignati A, Colombo L. Assessment of female fertility and carcinogenesis after iodine-131 therapy for differentiated thyroid carcinoma. J Nucl Med 1995;36(1):21–27.

69. Shepler TR, Sherman SI, Faustina MM, Busaidy NL, Ahmadi MA, Esmaeli B. Naso-lacrimal duct obstruction associated with radioactive iodine therapy for thyroid carcinoma. Ophthal Plast Reconstr Surg 2003;19(6):479–481.

70. Seidlin SM, Siegel E, Melamed S, Yalow AA. Occurrence of myeloid leukemia in patients with metastatic thyroid carcinoma following prolonged massive radioiodine therapy. Bull NY Acad Med 1955;31(5):410.

71. Seidlin SM, Siegal E, Yalow AA, Melamed S. Acute myeloid leukemia following prolonged iodine-131 therapy for metastatic thyroid carcinoma. Science 1956; 123(3201):800–801.

72. Pochin E. Long-term hazards of radioiodine treatment of thyroid carcinoma. In: Hedinger C, ed. Thyroid Cancer. UICC Monograph Series. Vol 12. Berlin: Springer-Verlag; 1969:293–304.

73. Bakheet SM, Powe J, Hammami MM. Unilateral radioiodine breast uptake. Clin Nucl Med 1998;23(3):170–171.

74. Bakheet SM, Hammami MM. Patterns of radioiodine uptake by the lactating breast. Eur J Nucl Med 1994;21(7):604–608.

75. Li CI, Rossing MA, Voigt LF, Daling JR. Multiple primary breast and thyroid cancers: role of age at diagnosis and cancer treatments (United States). Cancer Causes Control 2000;11(9):805–811.

76. Chen AY, Levy L, Goepfert H, Brown BW, Spitz MR, Vassilopoulou-Sellin R. The development of breast carcinoma in women with thyroid carcinoma. Cancer 2001;92(2):225–231.

77. Adjadj E, Rubino C, Shamsaldim A, Le MG, Schlumberger M, de Vathaire F. The risk of multiple primary breast and thyroid carcinomas. Cancer 2003;98(6):1309–1317.

78. Glanzmann C. Subsequent malignancies in patients treated with 131-iodine for thyroid cancer. Strahlenther Onkol 1992;168(6):337–343.

79. Schlumberger M, De Vathaire F, Ceccarelli C, et al. Exposure to radioactive iodine-131 for scintigraphy or therapy does not preclude pregnancy in thyroid cancer patients. J Nucl Med 1996;37(4):606–612.

80. Vini L, Hyer S, Al-Saadi A, Pratt B, Harmer C. Prognosis for fertility and ovarian function after treatment with radioiodine for thyroid cancer. Postgrad Med J 2002;78(916):92–93.

81. Pacini F, Gasperi M, Fugazzola L, et al. Testicular function in patients with differentiated thyroid carcinoma treated with radioiodine. J Nucl Med 1994;35(9):1418–1422.

82. Hyer S, Vini L, O'Connell M, Pratt B, Harmer C. Testicular dose and fertility in men following I(131) therapy for thyroid cancer. Clin Endocrinol (Oxf) 2002;56(6):755–758.

83. Ceccarelli C, Bencivelli W, Morciano D, Pinchera A, Pacini F. 131I therapy for differentiated thyroid cancer leads to an earlier onset of menopause: results of a retrospective study. J Clin Endocrinol Metab 2001;86(8):3512–3515.

84. Rall JE, Alpers JB, Lewallen CG, Sonenberg M, Berman M, Rawson RW. Radiation pneumonitis and fibrosis: a complication of radioiodine treatment of pulmonary metastases from cancer of the thyroid. J Clin Endocrinol Metab 1957;17(11):1263–1276.

85. Ali N, Sebastian C, Foley RR, et al. The management of differentiated thyroid cancer using 123I for imaging to assess the need for 131I therapy. Nucl Med Commun 2006;27(2):165–169.

86. Carr EA Jr, Dingledine WS, Beierwaltes WH. Premature resort to x-ray therapy: a common error in treatment of carcinoma of the thyroid gland. J Lancet 1958;78(11):478–483.

87. Wong JB, Kaplan MM, Meyer KB, Pauker SG. Ablative radioactive iodine therapy for apparently localized thyroid carcinoma. A decision analytic perspective. Endocrinol Metab Clin North Am 1990;19(3):741–760.

88. Sawka AM, Thephamongkhol K, Brouwers M, Thabane L, Browman G, Gerstein HC. Clinical review 170: a systematic review and metaanalysis of the effectiveness of radioactive iodine remnant ablation for well-differentiated thyroid cancer. J Clin Endocrinol Metab 2004;89(8):3668–3676.

89. Mazzaferri E. A randomized trial of remnant ablation—in search of an impossible dream? J Clin Endocrinol Metab 2004;89(8):3662–3664.

90. Haugen BR. Initial treatment of differentiated thyroid carcinoma. Rev Endocr Metab Disord 2000;1(3):139–145.

91. Taylor T, Specker B, Robbins J, et al. Outcome after treatment of high-risk papillary and non-Hürthle-cell follicular thyroid carcinoma. Ann Intern Med 1998;129(8):622–627.

92. Cunningham MP, Duda RB, Recant W, Chmiel JS, Sylvester JA, Fremgen A. Survival discriminants for differentiated thyroid cancer. Am J Surg 1990;160(4):344–347.

93. Hay ID, Thompson GB, Grant CS, et al. Papillary thyroid carcinoma managed at the Mayo Clinic during six decades (1940–1999): temporal trends in initial therapy and long-term outcome in 2444 consecutively treated patients. World J Surg 2002;26(8):879–885.

94. Van Wyngaarden K, McDougall IR. Is serum thyroglobulin a useful marker for thyroid cancer in patients who have not had ablation of residual thyroid tissue? Thyroid 1997;7(3):343–346.

95. Kalinyak JE, McDougall IR. Whole-body scanning with radionuclides of iodine and the controversy of thyroid stunning. Nucl Med Commun 2004;25:883–889.

96. Park H, Perkins OW, Edmondson JW, Schnute RB, Manatunga A. Influence of diagnostic radioiodines on the uptake of ablative dose of iodine-131. Thyroid 1994;4:49–54.

97. Muratet J, Daver A, Minier JF, Larra F. Influence of scanning doses of iodine-131 on subsequent first ablative treatment outcome in patients operated on for differentiated thyroid carcinoma. J Nucl Med 1998;39:1546–1550.

98. Leger F, Izembart M, Dagousset F, et al. Decreased uptake of therapeutic doses of iodine-131 after 185-MBq iodine-131 diagnostic imaging for thyroid remnants in differentiated thyroid carcinoma. Eur J Nucl Med 1998;25:242–246.

99. Cholewinski SP, Yoo KS, Klieger PS, O'Mara RE. Absence of thyroid stunning after diagnostic whole-body scanning with 185 MBq 131I. J Nucl Med 2000;41(7):1198–1202.

100. Sisson J, Jamadar DA, Kazerooni EA, Giordano TJ, Carey JE, Spaulding SA. Treatment of micronodular metastases of papillary thyroid cancer: are tumors too small for effective irradiation from radioiodine? Thyroid 1999;8:215–221.

101. Pineda J, Lee T, Ain K, Reynolds JC, Robbins J. Iodine-131 therapy for thyroid cancer patients with elevated thyroglobulin and negative diagnostic scan. J Clin Endocrinol Metab 1995;80:1488–1492.

102. Schlumberger M, Mancusi F, Baudin E, Pacini F. 131I therapy for elevated thyroglobulin levels. Thyroid 1997;7:273–276.

103. McDougall IR. Management of thyroglobulin positive/whole-body scan negative: is Tg positive/131I therapy useful? J Endocrinol Invest 2001;24(3):194–198.

104. Fatourechi V, Hay ID, Javedan H, Wiseman GA, Mullan BP, Gorman CA. Lack of impact of radioiodine therapy in Tg-positive, diagnostic whole-body scan-negative patients with follicular cell-derived thyroid cancer. J Clin Endocrinol Metab 2002; 87(4):1521–1526.

105. Wang W, Larson SM, Tuttle RM, et al. Resistance of [18f]-fluorodeoxyglucose-avid metastatic thyroid cancer lesions to treatment with high-dose radioactive iodine. Thyroid 2001;11(12):1169–1175.

106. Karwowski J, Jeffrey RB, McDougall IR, Weigel RJ. Intraoperative ultrasonography improves identification of recurrent thyroid cancer. Surgery 2002;132:924–928.

107. Smit JW, Links TP, Hew JM, Goslings BM, Vielvoye GJ, Vermey A. [Embolization of skeletal metastases in patients with differentiated thyroid carcinoma]. Ned Tijdschr Geneeskd 2000;144(29):1406–1410.

108. van Herle AJA, Agatep ML, Padua DN 3rd, et al. Effects of 13 cis-retinoic acid on growth and differentiation of human follicular carcinoma cells (UCLA RO 82 W-1) in vitro. J Clin Invest 1990;71:755–763.

109. Simon D, Korber C, Krausch M, et al. Clinical impact of retinoids in redifferentiation therapy of advanced thyroid cancer: final results of a pilot study. Eur J Nucl Med Mol Imaging 2002;29(6):775–782.

110. Gruning T, Tiepolt C, Zophel K, Bredow J, Kropp J, Franke WG. Retinoic acid for redifferentiation of thyroid cancer—does it hold its promise? Eur J Endocrinol 2003;148(4):395–402.

111. Schraube P, Kimmig B, zum Winkel K. [Lithium as an adjuvant in the radioiodine therapy of thyroid cancer]. Nuklearmedizin 1984;23(3):151–154.

112. Koong SS, Reynolds JC, Movius EG, et al. Lithium as a potential adjuvant to 131I therapy of metastatic, well differentiated thyroid carcinoma. J Clin Endocrinol Metab 1999;84(3):912–916.

6. Differentiated Thyroid Cancer: Rare Clinical Situations

Familial Differentiated Thyroid Cancer

The significance of differentiated thyroid cancers demonstrating familial aggregations has only recently been generally accepted.[1,2] Familial thyroid cancer could be the result of chance, a common etiologic factor, or genetic. When there are three first-degree relatives with thyroid cancer, chance becomes increasingly unlikely.[3,4] At this time, there is no single causal gene. Familial differentiated thyroid cancer is thought by some to have a poorer prognosis.[2,5] In 258 families with two or more differentiated thyroid cancers compared with 6200 sporadic cases, multifocal disease was present in 40.7% versus 29.8%, and recurrence rate was 16.3% versus 9.6%.[6] My experience with 34 families with two or more cases is that the outcome is similar to sporadic cancer. Associated disorders include familial adenomatous polyposis, Cowden's disease, Gardner's syndrome, and Peutz-Jeghers' syndrome. Total thyroidectomy is advised and when the cancer is large and there is local invasion or nodal or distant metastases, ^{131}I treatment is recommended. Patients would be followed by periodic clinical examination, measurement of thyroglobulin (Tg) and thyroid function, and imaging test such as ^{123}I scintigraphy and ultrasound. In families with three or more cancers, prospective evaluation of other members by careful palpation of the thyroid should be conducted.

Thyroid Cancer and End-Stage Renal Disease

Rarely a patient with end-stage renal disease has thyroid cancer and it is possible to treat a patient on dialysis with [131]I.[7] Each hemodialysis results in a reduction of about 60% of the radioactivity. Using dosimetric calculations based on whole-body measurements of a tracer of ^{131}I before and after two sets of dialysis dosimetry, we treated a patient on two occasions with 100 mCi (3.7 GBq). Other clinicians also recommend dosimetry.[8] In contrast, peritoneal dialysis reduces the radiation by only 10%–20% and the safe administered dose is 20–25 mCi (740–925 MBq).[9] Thus, the situation differs regarding whether the patient is on mechanical or peritoneal dialysis and dosimetry; therefore, ensuring that the blood and marrow are not exposed to an excessive absorbed dose is strongly advised in both.

Differentiated Thyroid Cancer Arising in Ectopic Sites

Cancer in Thyroglossal Tract

Thyroid cancers can occur in thyroglossal cysts and in ectopic thyroid. Cancers in thyroglossal cysts are more common but these are still quite rare. Heshmati et al.[10] in their 1997 report of 12 patients indicated that there were fewer than 200 cases in the literature. Thyroglossal duct cancer is slightly more common in women and the average age of the patients is about 40–45 years. A recent report of the literature identified only 17 cancers in patients younger than 16 years of age contrasting with the 7% incidence in thyroglossal remnants.[11] Approximately 80%–90% of thyroglossal cyst cancers are papillary.[12] The correct operation for thyroglossal cyst whether benign or malignant is the Sistrunk procedure. This involves removal of the thyroglossal tract from the base of the tongue, a small segment on the hyoid bone, the cyst, and the tract down to the isthmus of the thyroid. Some believe that the Sistrunk procedure is sufficient therapy for thyroglossal cyst cancer but others recommend total thyroidectomy as well.[13] The cancer might have arisen in the thyroid and migrated along the thyroglossal duct into the cyst. When a thyroglossal cyst is found to contain a cancer, clinical examination and ultrasound of the thyroid are recommended to ensure there is no mass in the thyroid. Then thyroidectomy may not be necessary and follow-up by clinical examination annually for several years is reasonable. When there is a thyroid mass, the gland should be removed, i.e., total thyroidectomy and Sistrunk procedure. Then treatment of residual functioning tissue with ^{131}I is advised. However, in practice, thyroglossal duct cancer is usually an unexpected finding on histologic examination of a surgically removed thyroglossal cyst and the decision regarding thyroidectomy is secondary. Distant metastases and death from this cancer are extremely rare.

Cancer in Lingual Thyroid

Lingual thyroid cancer is very rare and a recent article identified only 28 cases.[14] The majority are follicular. When the lingual thyroid does not shrink after treatment with L-thyroxine or when the lesion is bleeding or ulcerated, a biopsy should be obtained. Lingual thyroid cancer is best treated by surgery. The correct surgical approach depends on the specific skills of the surgeon and the size and stage of the cancer. The goal of surgery is to remove all normal and malignant thyroid cells but when the cancer is large and invasive the procedure will be damaging to the tongue. The ectopic tissue is usually the only site of functioning thyroid. After surgical excision, there is a role for scanning with radioiodine using the techniques discussed previously.[15] Abnormal uptake can be treated with [131]I. The patient should then be treated for life with an adequate dose of levothyroxine and followed with the same protocol for intrathyroidal cancer by scintiscan, ultrasound, and measurement of Tg and thyroid function.

Malignant Struma Ovarii

Struma ovarii is a teratoma in which more than 50% is thyroid. Struma ovarii can be asymptomatic, it can present as an ovarian mass, it is a rare cause of thyrotoxicosis, and it can produce ascites.[16] A struma ovarii should be removed surgically and it is usually a postoperative histologic diagnosis. Most struma ovarii are benign and to establish that one is malignant some authorities require evidence of capsular or vascular invasion, peritoneal involvement, or metastases. The intermingling of tissues of different lineage is insufficient evidence to determine the lesion is malignant. About 70% of malignant struma ovarii are papillary cancers or variants and 30% follicular.[17] Follicular cancers are more likely to metastasize widely and they have the same predilection for the skeleton and lungs.[18,19] There is a higher probability of liver metastases with malignant struma ovarii compared with primary thyroid cancer.[20]

When distant metastases containing cancerous thyroid are identified, it is important to exclude thyroid cancer in the cervical position as the site of the primary lesion. If this is confirmed, the struma ovarii has to be malignant. This also excludes the very rare chance of a primary thyroid cancer metastasizing to the ovary. When the malignant struma ovarii has been completely removed surgically, there is no need for additional surgery on the thyroid and there is no need for radical hysterectomy and bilateral oophorectomy.[21] Distant metastases from a malignant struma ovarii are rare. None of 13 patients in one series developed metastases.[22] Pardo-Mindan and Vazquez[23] identified 18 reports in the world literature. My colleagues and I have added two others.[20,24] A 42-year-old woman presented with spinal cord compression at the level of T2; the other patient had widespread hepatic metastases identified when she was investigated for severe abdominal pain. When there are distant metastases, it is important to remove the thyroid for two reasons: first, to ensure there is no evidence of primary thyroid cancer,[24,25] and second, it makes treatment of functioning metastases with ^{131}I possible. Therefore, a patient with functioning metastases is treated by surgery of the primary lesion, the thyroid, and bulky metastases followed by [131]I.

Variants of Papillary Cancer

Follicular Variant of Papillary Cancer

Approximately 10% of papillary cancers are of the follicular variant. Eighty percent of the cancer should be follicular in appearance. The nuclear features are identical to papillary cancer and this establishes that the lesion is papillary and not follicular cancer. There is no prognostic significance of this pathologic diagnosis and its natural history is similar to the standard papillary thyroid cancer and its management is exactly the same.

Tall Cell Variant of Papillary Cancer

Tall cell papillary cancer is a pathologic variant that is more aggressive clinically. The cells are at least twice as long as their breadth. There is usually local invasion, and nodal metastases. Recurrences and a higher death rate are anticipated. The patients are older than for standard papillary cancer and the cancer is larger. The first investigation should be fine needle aspiration (FNA). Therapy is designed to remove all cancer. Thyroidectomy should be complete and abnormal lymph nodes removed by modified neck dissection. Residual functioning thyroid should be ablated with [131]I. Cancerous tall cells often lack sodium iodide symporter and there can be residual disease that is not identified on scan. The patient is "scan negative, Tg positive." There is a role for positron emission tomography (PET) or PET/computed tomography (CT) to identify the site of Tg production.

Columnar Cell Variant of Papillary Cancer

This cancer is also associated with a bad prognosis. The cancerous cells look like respiratory epithelium. The pathologic hallmarks are columnar shape of the follicular cells, nuclear pseudostratification, prominent papulations, cytoplasmic clearing, and subnuclear vacuolization. There can be a question whether the cancer is actually a metastasis from adenocarcinoma of the nasopharynx, lung, ovary, or colon, but columnar cell cancer stains positively for Tg and thyroid transcription factor-1. The patient is usually elderly and has a new thyroid nodule that is hard and irregular. Total thyroidectomy rather than lobectomy is undertaken. This is a rare variant and there are only a few reports of diagnosis by FNA. Patients often have metastases at presentation. [131]I treatment to ablate residual thyroid and functioning metastases is recommended. This cancer has a significantly poorer prognosis than papillary thyroid cancer and many of the patient reports end with death.

Solid (Trabecular) Variant of Papillary Cancer

This cancer consists of solid nests of thyroid cells and 70% of the cancer should be solid for this designation. The nuclear features are typical of papillary cancer including nuclear clearing, pseudoinclusions, and nuclear grooves. This pathologic appearance has been described in children exposed to radioactive fallout from Chernobyl. There is a strong correlation with *RET/PTC3* rearrangement in these children.[26] The patient is usually a child or young adult, with a 3:1 ratio of women to men. Once the diagnosis is established by FNA, the patient should undergo a total thyroidectomy with removal of abnormal nodes. Postoperative treatment with ^{131}I to ablate residual thyroid and metastases is recommended. This variant is more aggressive than classical papillary cancer and there is higher probability of distant metastases. Ninety percent survival after an average follow-up of 18.7 years has been reported.[27]

Insular Cancer (Poorly Differentiated Cancer)

Insular cancer lies pathologically and clinically between differentiated thyroid cancers and anaplastic cancer. This is also called poorly differentiated thyroid cancer. And occasionally, "poorly differentiated insular cancer." About 1%–4% of thyroid cancers are of this variety. The patients are usually 40–60 years of age but there are reports of children as young as 10 years and adolescents with this diagnosis. There is approximately a 2:1 ratio of women to men. The cancer is often large and causes local pressure on breathing and swallowing. FNA is advised and although a diagnosis of cancer is established the specific diagnosis of insular cancer can be difficult because of nonspecific cytopathologic findings. When nests of cells 0.2–0.4 mm in diameter are noted on a cytology specimen, insular cancer is likely.[28] Distant metastases to the lung or bones can be the presenting feature. The odds ratio of developing distant metastases when there is an insular component is 17 ($P < .0001$).[29] The cancers are large with a high incidence of capsular and vascular invasion. One study in 46 specimens with insular features demonstrated a mutation in the cancer suppressor $p53$ gene.[30] Retrospective reviews of some anaplastic cancers can result in reclassification as poorly differentiated insular cancers. The standard therapy is total thyroidectomy, removal of suspicious cervical lymph nodes, and postoperative radioiodine [131]I. A proportion of insular cancers and their metastases do not trap iodine. However, there are rare reports of distant metastases, including skeletal metastases, demonstrating uptake. When there is uncertainty about the stage or extent of disease, ^{18}F-fluorodeoxyglucose (FDG) PET/CT scan should be considered.

Patients with insular cancer of the thyroid have a prognosis that is worse than papillary or follicular cancer but better than anaplastic cancer. Because of the aggressive nature of the cancer and its potential for local and distant spread, there is an argument for more complete surgery and larger doses of ^{131}I to try to remove all cancer cells at the time of presentation.

Variants of Follicular Cancer: Hürthle Cell Cancer

Hürthle cells are follicular cells with abundant cytoplasmic mitochondria.[31] They can be identified in Hashimoto's thyroiditis, Graves' disease, in addition to neoplasia. The cells look active but paradoxically they do not trap iodine. The patient is older (average 50–60 years), the cancer is more aggressive, and its management different. Therefore, many authorities classify Hürthle cell cancers separately from differentiated thyroid cancer.[32] Controversies are how to distinguish Hürthle cell carcinoma from Hürthle cell adenoma and how to treat and follow patients with proven Hürthle cell cancer. To establish that the lesion is cancer, there has to be evidence of regional, or distant metastases, or pathologically the lesion should demonstrate angioinvasion, or capsular invasion. One group use three clinical categories: widely invasive cancer, minimally invasive cancer, and tumors of unknown malignant behavior.[33] These cannot be differentiated cytologically. The definitive diagnosis depends on histopathology but even then there can be differences of opinion. The differentiation of benign from malignant Hürthle cell neoplasm is not always straightforward and a second pathologic opinion is warranted in borderline cases.

The patient presents with a nodule. There is a 2:1 ratio of women to men. In one series, 9% of the patients were diagnosed from a distant metastasis.[34] Free T4 and thyrotropin should be ordered and FNA undertaken. The FNA report will generally be worded, "Hürthle cell neoplasm, it is not possible to differentiate Hürthle cell adenoma from Hürthle cell carcinoma: recommend surgical excision." The dilemma is whether to advise a lobectomy, versus total thyroidectomy. The authorities from the University of Michigan recommend when the lesion is >2 cm, it should be considered malignant and the entire thyroid be removed.[35] This is based on finding metastases on follow-up in 3 of 26 patients whose pathology was judged to be benign but who had large lesions. Intraoperative frozen section only helps determine the extent of operation in 1 of 5 patients.[36] This frequently results in only a lobe being removed and the need to complete the thyroidectomy when the final pathology confirms features of cancer. [131]I is advised for patients with large cancers, widely invasive cancers, those with high Tg values after surgery, and those with local invasion. However, metastases from Hürthle cell cancer seldom trap radioiodine; therefore, this therapy is generally of no benefit when the cancer has spread. The purpose of radioiodine is to remove functioning thyroid, and then Tg should be measured. If Tg is undetectable, it is likely the patient has been cured. The higher the Tg value after thyroidectomy and ^{131}I, the more likely there is residual disease or distant metastases. [18]FDG-PET/CT has excellent sensitivity for identifying metastases.[37] When PET is not available, ^{99m}Tc-sestamibi can be useful. Once the site of metastatic cancer is identified, a decision about surgery versus external radiation can be made based on the location of the lesion. Cancers larger than 4 cm with extensive capsular and angioinvasion, lymph node and distant metastases, have a poor prognosis. Older patients also have a poorer prognosis.

References

1. Burgess J, Duffield A, Wilkinson SJ, et al. Two families with an autosomal dominant inheritance pattern for papillary carcinoma of the thyroid. J Clin Endocrinol Metab 1997;82:345–348.

2. Loh KC. Familial nonmedullary thyroid carcinoma: a meta-review of case series. Thyroid 1997;7(1):107–113.

3. Houlston R. Genetic predisposition to non-medullary thyroid cancer. Nucl Med Commun 1998;19:911–913.

4. Malchoff CD, Malchoff DM. Familial nonmedullary thyroid carcinoma. Semin Surg Oncol 1999;16(1):16–18.

5. Alsanea O, Wada N, Ain K, et al. Is familial non-medullary thyroid carcinoma more aggressive than sporadic thyroid cancer? A multicenter series. Surgery 2000;128(6): 1043–1050; discussion 1050–1051.

6. Uchino S, Noguchi S, Kawamoto H, Yamashita H, Watanabe S, Shuto S. Familial nonmedullary thyroid carcinoma characterized by multifocality and a high recurrence rate in a large study population. World J Surg 2002;26(8):897–902.

7. Mello AM, Isaacs R, Petersen J, Kronenberger S, McDougall IR. Management of thyroid papillary carcinoma with radioiodine in a patient with end stage renal disease on hemodialysis. Clin Nucl Med 1994;19(9):776–781.

8. Holst JP, Burman KD, Atkins F, Umans JG, Jonklaas J. Radioiodine therapy for thyroid cancer and hyperthyroidism in patients with end-stage renal disease on hemodialysis. Thyroid 2005;15(12):1321–1331.

9. Kaptein EM, Levenson H, Siegel ME, Gadallah M, Akmal M. Radioiodine dosimetry in patients with end-stage renal disease receiving continuous ambulatory peritoneal dialysis therapy. J Clin Endocrinol Metab 2000;85(9):3058–3064.

10. Heshmati HM, Fatourechi V, van Heerden JA, Hay ID, Goellner JR. Thyroglossal duct carcinoma: report of 12 cases. Mayo Clin Proc 1997;72(4):315–319.

11. Peretz A, Leiberman E, Kapelushnik J, Hershkovitz E. Thyroglossal duct carcinoma in children: case presentation and review of the literature. Thyroid 2004;14(9): 777–785.

12. Seoane JM, Cameselle-Teijeiro J, Romero MA. Poorly differentiated oxyphilic (Hürthle cell) carcinoma arising in lingual thyroid: a case report and review of the literature. Endocr Pathol 2002;13(4):353–360.

13. Miccoli P, Minuto MN, Galleri D, Puccini M, Berti P. Extent of surgery in thyroglossal duct carcinoma: reflections on a series of eighteen cases. Thyroid 2004;14(2): 121–123.

14. Massine RE, Durning SJ, Koroscil TM. Lingual thyroid carcinoma: a case report and review of the literature. Thyroid 2001;11(12):1191–1196.

15. Mill WA, Gowing NF, Reeves B, Smithers DW. Carcinoma of the lingual thyroid treated with radioactive iodine. Lancet 1959;1(7063):76–79.

16. Kempers RD, Dockerty MB, Hoffman DL, Bartholomew LG. Struma ovarii—ascitic, hyperthyroid, and asymptomatic syndromes. Ann Intern Med 1970;72(6):883–893.

17. Navarro MD, Tan MA, Lovecchio JL, Hajdu SI. Case report: malignant struma ovarii. Ann Clin Lab Sci 2004;34(1):107–112.

18. Tokuda Y, Hatayama T, Sakoda K. Metastasis of malignant struma ovarii to the cranial vault during pregnancy. Neurosurgery 1993;33(3):515–518.

19. Checrallah A, Medlej R, Saade C, Khayat G, Halaby G. Malignant struma ovarii: an unusual presentation. Thyroid 2001;11(9):889–892.

20. McDougall I. Metastatic struma ovarii: the burden of truth. Clin Nucl Med 2006; 31:321–324.

21. Nahn PA, Robinson E, Strassman M. Conservative therapy for malignant struma ovarii. A case report. J Reprod Med 2002;47(11):943–945.

22. Devaney K, Snyder R, Norris HJ, Tavassoli FA. Proliferative and histologically malignant struma ovarii: a clinicopathologic study of 54 cases. Int J Gynecol Pathol 1993;12(4):333–343.

23. Pardo-Mindan FJ, Vazquez JJ. Malignant struma ovarii. Light and electron microscopic study. Cancer 1983;51(2):337–343.

24. McDougall IR, Krasne D, Hanbery JW, Collins JA. Metastatic malignant struma ovarii presenting as paraparesis from a spinal metastasis. J Nucl Med 1989;30(3): 407–411.

25. Chan SW, Farrell KE. Metastatic thyroid carcinoma in the presence of struma ovarii. Med J Aust 2001;175(7):373–374.

26. Nikiforov Y, Gnepp DR, Fagin JA. Thyroid lesions in children and adolescents after the Chernobyl disaster: implications for the study of radiation tumorigenesis. J Clin Endocrinol Metab 1996;81(1):9–14.

27. Nikiforov YE, Erickson LA, Nikiforova MN, Caudill CM, Lloyd RV. Solid variant of papillary thyroid carcinoma: incidence, clinical-pathologic characteristics, molecular analysis, and biologic behavior. Am J Surg Pathol 2001;25(12):1478–1484.

28. Kuhel WI, Kutler DI, Santos-Buch CA. Poorly differentiated insular thyroid carcinoma. A case report with identification of intact insulae with fine needle aspiration biopsy. Acta Cytol 1998;42(4):991–997.

29. Decaussin M, Bernard MH, Adeleine P, et al. Thyroid carcinoma with distant metastases. A review of 11 cases with emphasis on the prognostic significance of the insular component. Am J Surg Pathol 2002;26:1007–1015.

30. Takeuchi Y, Daa T, Kashima K, Yokoyama S, Nakayama I, Noguchi S. Mutations of p53 in thyroid carcinoma with an insular component. Thyroid 1999;9(4):377–381.

31. Tallini G, Carcangiu ML, Rosai J. Oncocytic neoplasms of the thyroid gland. Acta Pathol Jpn 1992;42(5):305–315.

32. Watson RG, Brennan MD, Goellner JR, van Heerden JA, McConahey WM, Taylor WF. Invasive Hürthle cell carcinoma of the thyroid: natural history and management. Mayo Clin Proc 1984;59(12):851–855.

33. Stojadinovic A, Ghossein RA, Hoos A, et al. Hürthle cell carcinoma: a critical histopathologic appraisal. J Clin Oncol 2001;19(10):2616–2625.

34. Lopez-Penabad L, Chiu AC, Hoff AO, et al. Prognostic factors in patients with Hürthle cell neoplasms of the thyroid. Cancer 2003;97(5):1186–1194.

35. Gundry SR, Burney RE, Thompson NW, Lloyd R. Total thyroidectomy for Hürthle cell neoplasm of the thyroid. Arch Surg 1983;118(5):529–532.

36. Dahl LD, Myssiorek D, Heller KS. Hürthle cell neoplasms of the thyroid. Laryngoscope 2002;112(12):2178–2180.

37. Plotkin M, Hautzel H, Krause BJ, et al. Implication of 2-[18]fluor-2-deoxyglucose positron emission tomography in the follow-up of Hürthle cell thyroid cancer. Thyroid 2002;12(2):155–161.

7. Differentiated Thyroid Cancer in Children

Thyroid cancer arising from the follicular cells in children is rare and few physicians have experience with its diagnosis and management. Also, few surgeons are trained in conducting thyroidectomies in children. There are some differences in thyroid cancer in children compared with adults. The cancers in pediatric patients are almost all papillary and more advanced. The primary cancer is often larger than in adults plus multifocality and local invasion are more common as are metastases to cervical lymph nodes and distant metastases to the lungs. The recurrence rate is also higher. Complications of treatment are more common and have to be lived with for many decades. The parents want to know the implications of the disease and treatments on longevity, fertility, and unborn grandchildren. The doctor needs to be constantly there for the patient and family. The role of radiation and genetics as causal factors was presented in Chapter 1.

Incidence

Approximately 7.5% of childhood cancers are thyroidal (1–3 per million children).[1] In 15–19 year olds, thyroid cancer ranks eighth but because there are 4 times as many women with this cancer, it is the second most common tumor in women of this age. In prepubertal children, there is a small excess of males.[2] My experience is with 71 children 20 years of age or younger (average 14.7 years). Fifty-three (75%) are women. Eleven patients were 10 years or younger. In the United Kingdom, only 154 cases of thyroid cancer were reported in children under the age of 15 years over 3 decades.

Presentation and Diagnosis

The cancer usually presents as a nodule in the thyroid or as metastases to cervical lymph nodes. Most pediatricians have never seen a patient with thyroid cancer but they all see many children with enlarged cervical nodes. Therefore, the likelihood that a child with a neck swelling has thyroid cancer is small and usually not considered. Thyroid nodules are rare in children but the risk of the nodule being a cancer is proportionately greater. An explanation for the more advanced disease in the pediatric patient is a delay in diagnosis.

Expeditious workup of a child with a thyroid nodule, an enlarging thyroid, or enlarged cervical lymph nodes should be stressed. The best investigation is fine needle aspiration (FNA) of the thyroid nodule, or lymph node.[3] Thyroid scintiscan is of almost no value in children with a thyroid nodule. Functioning nodules are very rare in children but they have a risk of being malignant.[4] Therefore, it does not matter whether the thyroid nodule is "hot" or "cold" on scan—the risk of cancer is there. In a multicenter study, the positive predictive value (PPV) of thyroid scintiscan was 12% and the negative predictive value (NPV) 68%.[5] The PPV for ultrasound was also low at 15%. In contrast, the PPV and NPV for FNA were 67% and 100%, respectively. FNA is accurate and the best single test to differentiate a benign from a malignant thyroid nodule. Thyroid ultrasound can help direct FNA. There is value of having a cytology technologist present during the procedure to stain the specimen and make a judgment that there are sufficient cells for interpretation. There should be no need for a repeat biopsy. If a second FNA is necessary, the results are improved with the use of ultrasound guidance. When the FNA is adequate and unequivocally benign and the nodule is not too large or clinically suspicious, it is reasonable to follow the patient. Annual clinic visits should be arranged for careful examination to determine the size and consistency of the nodule and whether there is any evidence of fixation. The cervical nodes should be examined. An ultrasound is valuable for an accurate measurement of length, width, and depth of the nodule. Any increase in size or change in characteristics of the nodule would be an indication for a repeat FNA and if the result is not benign the patient is referred to a skilled surgeon.

Most pediatric thyroid cancers are papillary with a high incidence of multifocality and invasion and lymph metastases, therefore total thyroidectomy is the optimal operation. A child with a thyroid nodule should not be referred for surgery without an FNA. However, in a multicenter study conducted by the Surgical Discipline Committee of the Children's Cancer Group, only 25% of 327 patients with thyroid cancer had a preoperative FNA.[6] The surgeon then has to rely on a frozen-section, intraoperative diagnosis to direct the extent of the operation and that interpretation is often indeterminate. This results in a decision to remove the lobe containing the nodule. When the definitive diagnosis of cancer is made several days later, the patient and family are advised that completion of thyroidectomy is required. The complication rate is higher in "redo" procedures. In contrast, when the diagnosis is established preoperatively, only one operation is necessary.

Occasionally there can be cancer, usually papillary in type within a thyroglossal duct cyst. Because fewer than 1% of thyroglossal cysts contain a cancer, the cost effectiveness of FNA in children is debatable. In a review of the world literature of cancer in thyroglossal duct cyst, there were only 17 patients under the age of 16.[7] This contrasts with the fact that thyroglossal cysts are the second most common cause of a nodule in the neck of children. When there is cancer, there is some debate whether the Sistrunk operation alone is sufficient or whether it should be coupled with thyroidectomy. The reasons for thyroidectomy are that there can be cancer in the thyroid in 30%–40%, nodal metastases cannot be treated with ^{131}I until the thyroid is removed and thyroglobulin (Tg) is not such a reliable tumor marker when the thyroid remains. When the cancer in the thyroglossal duct is small and fully excised and when there is no palpable mass or abnormality on ultrasound of the thyroid, the Sistrunk operation is sufficient and the long-term results are excellent. A large, invasive thyroglossal duct cancer, the presence of a thyroid mass, or metastases in cervical nodes dictate that thyroidectomy is also required.

Pathology

In regions of high intake of dietary iodine, 85%–95% of thyroid cancers are papillary, and in iodine-deficient regions, this decreases to 60%–80%. At Stanford, 65 of 71 (91%) cancers in pediatric patients are papillary. The cancers are frequently multifocal. The average size is 3–4 cm.[6] Local invasion is common and lymph node metastases are found in more than 50% of patients. Distant metastases are reported in about 20%, most often to the lungs. In my experience, 76% had lymph node metastases and 34% pulmonary involvement. The histologic type of cancer in those exposed to nuclear fallout is commonly the solid variant of papillary cancer, which is more aggressive and there are reports of children dying from this cancer.[8] When a patient has had thyroidectomy and is referred for a consultation or for postoperative ^{131}I, it is important to review the pathology slides to confirm the diagnosis and define the size of the cancer, invasion, and identify any unusual histopathology. Very rarely, poorly differentiated cancer such as insular or anaplastic occurs in a child.[9]

Treatment

Total (near total) thyroidectomy, with removal of abnormal lymph nodes, is critical. In selected patients, ^{131}I is prescribed after the operation and thyroid hormone is prescribed for life.

Surgery

A skilled surgeon who can remove the thyroid in a child without producing complications is important. Retrospective studies show a higher recurrence rate after lobectomy.[10,11] Complications of surgery include damage to the recurrent laryngeal nerves, the superior laryngeal nerve, parathyroids, and in rare situations the spinal accessory nerve or the cervical sympathetic nerve. Between 10%–20% of pediatric patients have surgical complications.[12,13] When the cancer is small and fully excised, lobectomy (plus isthmusectomy) might suffice.[14] However, the data presented above indicate that many cancers are multifocal and many patients have lymph node and pulmonary metastases. Local recurrence is more likely and treatment of metastases with ^{131}I is difficult when there is a lobe of normal thyroid. One study reevaluated 47 children from Belarus whose parents desired a second opinion in Pisa, Italy.[15] Based on pathology and scintigraphic data, residual or metastatic thyroid cancer was identified in 61% of these patients. These data argue for a more complete primary operation by a skilled and experienced surgeon.

Thyroid Hormone

Thyroid hormone will be required for life. It is difficult for a child to be compulsive about taking a pill daily. The need must be reinforced at each clinic visit. It is impracticable to expect a child, or adolescent, to ingest thyroid hormone 1 hour before breakfast recognizing that food has an effect on absorption. The correct dose of L-thyroxine can be determined by testing thyroid function and adjusting the dose as necessary. Children require a higher dose than adults relative to their weight. The dose of L-thyroxine necessary to keep thyrotropin (TSH) at the low end of the range is close to 1 µg/lb. body weight. The importance of measuring serum TSH is stressed.

Radioiodine

Most authorities treat with ^{131}I after surgery.[16] In contrast, physicians at the Mayo Clinic do not recommend ^{131}I and rely on surgery and thyroid hormone.[17] They demonstrated an excellent outcome in 58 children of whom only 17% received postoperative [131]I. Eighty-six percent with pulmonary metastases were treated with [131]I. Ten of the patients that I have managed were not treated with radioiodine but they had early disease. The differences in opinion about ^{131}I are in part the result of the paradoxic presentation versus course of the cancer. The disease is advanced but children do not die from this cancer. When the cancer is <1.5 cm, single, noninvasive, and fully excised by an appropriate operation, there is no evidence that ^{131}I will reduce the recurrence rate, or improve survival.

When a decision is made to consider ^{131}I, the protocol is to withdraw thyroid hormone (thyroxine) for 4 weeks, or to wait 4 weeks from the time of thyroidectomy. It is very helpful to meet with the patient and parents to discuss the protocol and to give time for the family to plan and have any questions answered. It is possible to engage the patient as well as the parents with all aspects of this treatment unless the child is very young. The planning includes not only the dates for scanning but also treatment. Most children tolerate hypothyroidism well but the symptoms they will experience should be discussed. A low iodine diet should be provided. This advises a list of foods that can be eaten and those that should be avoided for 2 weeks before and through testing and treatment. The diet available from www.thyca.org is helpful. After 4 weeks, blood is drawn for measurement of TSH, Tg, and in women after menarche a pregnancy test. I arrange treatment on the same day as the diagnostic scan. Therefore, when the patient needs to be admitted to hospital, the room is available, the necessary authorizations from the insurance company are in place, and radiation safety officers informed. Some physicians proceed straight to ^{131}I treatment but most authorities obtain a whole-body scan with a diagnostic dose of radioiodine to identify the extent of residual disease. Historically, ^{131}I was and still is prescribed for the diagnostic scan. The usual dose is 37–155 MBq (1–5 mCi). In the past, I used 37–74 MBq (1–2 mCi) and scanned after 48–72 hours. Some experts are concerned that diagnostic ^{131}I might cause "stunning," meaning that the radiation delivered to the thyroid by the diagnostic dose of ^{131}I could cause sufficient cellular damage that the therapeutic dose of ^{131}I would not be trapped, or have less effect.[18] I did not find that, provided the dose of ^{131}I was 74 MBq (2 mCi) or less and the treatment was administered as soon after diagnostic scanning as possible.[19] More recently, several groups have recommended ^{123}I that emits only photons and subjects the patient and thyroid to less radiation than [131]I.[20,21] [123]I images are superior and can be extended to 48 hours when 4–5 mCi (148–185 MBq) is administered (Figure 7.1). The diagnostic scan allows the amount of residual thyroid to be determined, and when adequate surgery has been conducted, it also allows functioning metastases to be identified. Therefore, the therapeutic dose can be prescribed with knowledge of this information. Those who proceed directly to therapy have to make an empiric judgment about what therapeutic dose to administer. Figure 7.2 is a posttherapy scan in a young patient who has pulmonary metastases but had no diagnostic scan and was treated elsewhere with a small dose of ^{131}I for "ablation" of residual thyroid. It was not successful. A diagnostic scan would likely have caused a larger therapy dose to be administered.

There is little in the literature about the specific dose of [131]I. Mazzaferri[22] recommends 1.1 GBq (30 mCi) for ablation of thyroid remnants. The same dose is recommended by Hung and Sarlis.[23] Others administer doses of 0.925–5.5 GBq [131]I (25–150 mCi) for ablation.[24] An average first dose of 2.5 ± 0.96 GBq (67.5 ± 26 mCi) was administered by Chow et al.[25] The dose should be related to the size of the patient, their age, and the extent of disease. In children of 80 pounds (36 kg), 1.1–2.8 GBq (30–75 mCi) would be reasonable. When there is local invasion or nodal metastases, the range of doses would be between 3.7–5.5 GBq (100–150 mCi) [131]I. In the case of pulmonary metastases, depending on size, 1.85–5.5 GBq (50–150 mCi), and for bone metastases that are uncommon in children, 3.7–7.4 GBq (100–200 mCi), are advised. For smaller and younger children, the administered dose would be reduced. Grigsby et al.[26] prescribed 0.74–1.48 GBq (20–40 mCi) in children 6 years of age or younger. One patient aged 7 years received 4.4 GBq (120 mCi) and the cumulative doses of ^{131}I in 46 patients ranged from 1.1 to 30 GBq (31–810 mCi). This was similar to the range of 0.74–21.5 GBq (20–580 mCi) in the report of Chow et al.[25] and the maximum cumulative dose of 32.7 GBq (885 mCi) administered by Haveman et al.[24] A series of patients with pulmonary metastases received cumulative doses of

Diagnostic I-123   3 days post therapy

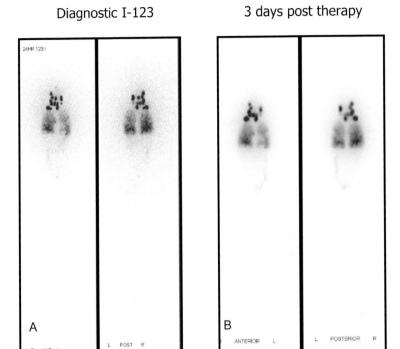

Figure 7.1. A Anterior and posterior whole-body scan made 24 hours after 74 mBq [123]I. It demonstrates multiple, functioning nodal metastases and diffuse, pulmonary metastases bilaterally. **B** Posttherapy scan demonstrating an identical pattern after treatment with [131]I.

4.6–38.7 GBq (125 mCi to 1.05 Ci).[27] In each of these reports, some patients received four or more treatments. Smaller doses were administered by other investigators, 0.37–1.85 GBq (10–50 mCi) for ablation and 1.85–3.7 GBq (50–100 mCi), to treat local or distant metastases.[28] It could be argued that the lower dose might work and when it does not a second dose can be prescribed. Most would advise the higher range with the concept of treating effectively on the first occasion. There is no controlled trial to judge the success of treatment. Some authorities place an upper limit of 22.2 MBq (600 mCi).[29] This is based on two concerns. First, that a higher dose could increase the risk of complications such as second cancers or marrow aplasia, and second, when this quantity has not worked, it is unlikely that an additional dose will. In patients with extensive metastases, it is reasonable to obtain objective data that the blood would not receive an absorbed dose of 200 rad (2 Gy) or that 80 mCi would be

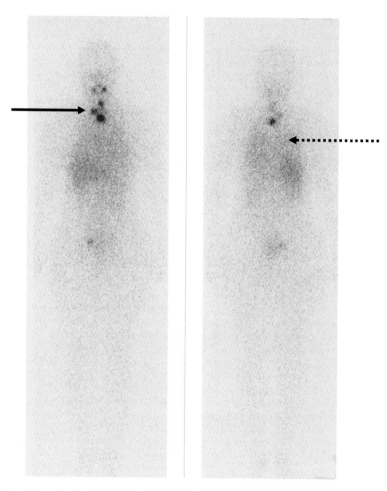

Figure 7.2. Posttherapy scan from an outside hospital processed 5 days after 1.85 GBq (50 mCi) [131]I. There are functioning nodal metastases (solid arrow) and diffuse lung uptake bilaterally from miliary metastases (dotted arrow). If a diagnostic scan had been obtained first, it is likely the patient would have been treated with a substantially larger dose.

retained in the lungs.[30] This can be obtained by using counts over the lung and whole body at 48 hours after the administration of the diagnostic tracer of radioiodine. Alternatively, the simple method of Sisson et al.[31] is to use a probe at a distance of 2.5 m and compare an early whole-body count at 1–2 hours and the 48-hour measurement.

There are important logistical issues. Usually, the diagnostic and therapeutic radioiodine is packaged in capsule form. Some small children have difficulty swallowing capsules. This should be assessed ahead of time and when necessary radioiodine can be obtained in liquid form. In adults, recombinant human TSH (rhTSH) has become a very important tool for conducting wholebody scintigraphy and measuring TSH-stimulated Tg.[32] rhTSH has not been approved for use in patients younger than 16 years of age and there are very few published data.[33]

Radiation Safety

For small doses of diagnostic ^{131}I and for ^{123}I, radiation safety issues are simple, but for therapeutic doses of ^{131}I, it is usually necessary to admit the patient to hospital. Readers should be cognizant of the regulations that apply in their country or state. In California, a patient can be released home when any one of the following pertains: 1) the patient receives 1.2 GBq (33 mCi) or less; 2) the emitted radiation is 7 mrem/h at 1 m or less; 3) no adult member of the public could receive 5 mSv (500 mrem) from the patient. The first two are easy to document. In the case of a patient receiving 3.7 MBq (100 mCi), the emitted radiation is approximately 20 mrem/h at 1 m at the time of treatment. If the patient is to be discharged, the treating physician has to document that the home situation would make it impossible for other members of the family to receive 5 mSv (500 mrem). The child would need to be an appropriate age and intellect so that an informed discussion about radiation safety can be conducted. The child should have a separate bedroom and preferably a separate bathroom. The distance and time (occupancy factor) other members of the house are from the patient must be predetermined. This allows a calculation about the decision to discharge the patient, or to admit to hospital. In one study, the radiation doses to family members and pets from radioactive patients were measured.[34] The mean dose to 64 family members was 0.24 mSv demonstrating that patients can be discharged after large doses of ^{131}I and the physician can comply with regulations. When there are young siblings or a pregnant relative in the home, or the living circumstances are cramped, it is preferable to admit the child to hospital. The treating physician and a member of the radiation safety group should review radiation safety issues with the nursing team.

Management After [131]I Treatment

The patient starts thyroid hormone and regular diet 24 hours after ^{131}I treatment. A posttherapy scan is obtained after 5–8 days. Occasionally, that scan can show better uptake in lesions and in rare cases it demonstrates new lesions. In my experience, when near total thyroidectomy is achieved and the patient studied by whole-body scan at the time TSH is >50 mU/L and on a low iodine diet, the posttreatment scan seldom increases the stage of disease but it confirms the therapy was concentrated and retained at the desired sites. At this appointment, the emitted radiation can be measured at a distance of a meter and this allows an informed decision about whether to maintain radiation safety regulations or to permit the child back to school, etc.

The patient returns after about 8 weeks for examination and for measurement of thyroid function, Tg, and if applicable calcium. Plans are made for a follow-up scan with measurement of stimulated Tg 6–12 months after the original therapy. It is usually more convenient to arrange this during school vacation because of the hypothyroidism, low iodine diet, absence from classes, and radioactivity (albeit relatively low dose). When the scan is negative and stimulated Tg low, I arrange follow-up at 6–month intervals. These visits include careful examination of the neck and measurement of thyroid function and Tg. Ultrasound of the neck can be obtained at intervals of 1–2 years. It is reasonable to rescan at 2 years. I think it is also reasonable provided the first scan and stimulated Tg are negative and nonstimulated Tg values are consistently undetectable to wait until 5 years to rescan and measure stimulated Tg. The fact that recurrences can occur is the driving force for long-term follow-up. When the follow-up scan and Tg are positive and there is no palpable disease, consideration should be given for additional [131]I. This is more likely in the case of distant metastases. Pulmonary lesions are usually micronodular in children and they can be imperceptible on chest roentgenogram and even computed tomography (CT). They can be identified on diagnostic whole-body scan and posttreatment scan, the latter having a higher sensitivity. Sisson et al.[35] comment that the majority of the energy of β particles of ^{131}I is deposited outside of millimeter-sized nodules. When the roentgenogram is normal and Tg low the benefit of repeated doses of ^{131}I in relation to risk decreases as the cumulative administered dose increases. Schlumberger[29] recommends a limit of 22.2 GBq (600 mCi).

False-Positive Scans

The normal distribution of radioiodine should be to residual thyroid and functioning metastases that are most often in regional cervical nodes and the lungs, salivary glands, stomach and intestines, and urinary tract. Diffuse uptake in the liver is seen on posttherapy scans made 4–8 days after treatment.[36] When a diagnostic scan shows accumulation of radioiodine in an unusual site, the physician should take time to determine whether this is a true or false positive. Carlisle et al.[37] have published an extensive list of false-positive findings including the references. The scan should be reviewed for technical qualities and compared with serum Tg because metastases are very uncommon when a stimulated Tg is undetectable. The most likely cause of a false positive is contaminant with radioactive saliva, mucus, or urine and sites that are superficial should be washed and the area rescanned.

Complications and Long-Term Problems After [131]I

An antiemetic can be prescribed when a large dose of ^{131}I is administered. Swelling of the salivary glands can occur but chronic salivary problems and permanent dryness of the mouth are rare in children. Concerns about fertility of the child and the effect of ^{131}I on future offspring are important. Two hundred seventy-six of 496 women under the age of 40 at the time of ^{131}I treatment gave birth to 427 children and there were no congenital abnormalities.[38] Only one woman who desired a baby was unable to conceive. In another retrospective review, the pregnancies and offspring of 70 women aged 15–36 years who were treated with a mean dose of 4.39 MBq (118 mCi) [131]I were evaluated.[39] There were two miscarriages and of 73 children, three had low birth weight and one had tetralogy of Fallot. The fertility and offspring of 627 women who were treated with ^{131}I were compared with 187 patients who did not receive [131]I.[40] There was no statistical difference in fertility, prematurity, or birth weights of the babies. Several other series confirm that it is safe for patients to conceive after an appropriate delay after [131]I (see below). My advice is that the patient does not become pregnant until a follow-up scan and measurement of Tg demonstrates successful treatment. Ayala et al.[41] described a higher incidence of problems within 1 year of ^{131}I suggesting that length of time is an appropriate delay. Dottorini et al.[42] described oligospermia in one patient who received 3.33 GBq (90 mCi). In contrast, Hyer et al.[43] evaluated fertility in 122 men who were younger than 40 years at the time of treatment with [131]I. Fifty-nine patients who wanted children, fathered 106 offspring, none of whom had a significant malformation. The testicular doses were 6.4 cGy after 3 GBq (6.4 rad after 81 mCi) and 14 cGy after 5.5 GBq (14 rad after 150 mCi). Follicle-stimulating hormone increased transiently but was normal after 9 months.

A pregnancy test must be obtained in any female who has reached menarche. Serum measurement is preferred, the result is available within an hour, and it is more sensitive than urinary testing. The topic is discussed in detail in the next chapter on thyroid cancer and pregnancy.

There is also concern that the radioiodine will cause or increase the risk of a second cancer. Most of the data relate to adults and overall the risk seems very small. One situation is of concern to me. When the patient is a postpubertal woman and there is uptake of the tracer of ^{123}I or ^{131}I in the breasts, I would defer radioiodine therapy. The breast is sensitive to radiation and there is evidence of an increase in breast cancer that could be attributed to this.

In patients with extensive pulmonary metastases, ^{131}I could damage normal lung surrounding the miliary cancer and cause fibrosis and reduced lung function as described in early reports.[44] More recent evidence indicates unchecked growth of the cancer is a more likely cause of difficulty breathing than the ^{131}I treatment.[27]

Controversies

The absence of a controlled study to determine whether ^{131}I improves the prognosis or reduces recurrences is a major limitation. The fact that an abnormality on scan can be shown to disappear on follow-up scan after radioiodine treatment is taken to mean success. Similarly, a reduction in Tg is accepted as evidence that cancer cells have been killed. However, the recurrence rate is substantial (see below). Up to 90% of children younger than 10 years at diagnosis have a recurrence.[45] Because of the small number of patients, there is little published about "stunning" of thyroid cells by diagnostic doses of ^{131}I in children. I found no evidence of this in children who had comparable diagnostic and posttherapy scans. There is no publication dealing specifically with Tg-positive scan-negative pediatric patients. The problem is the same as in the adult. Should the patient be monitored without intervention, should a large dose of ^{131}I be administered, or should other tests such as [18]fluorodeoxyglucose (FDG) positron emission tomography (PET)/CT scan be conducted? The origin of Tg could be in miliary lesions in the lungs and when they were identified on prior diagnostic and posttherapy scans, it is reasonable to administer one additional therapy dose in the hope that the cells will trap enough ^{131}I to be killed. When a prior posttreatment scan was negative, it is hard to argue in favor of another large dose. At the time of writing, there are no articles on [18]FDG PET/CT in the management of thyroid cancer in children. My experience with PET/CT in children with thyroid cancer is limited to four patients and therefore cannot determine policy. Lesions less than 4–5 mm are unlikely to be identified. Therefore, when a posttreatment scan and PET scan (and ultrasound of the neck) are negative, waiting and monitoring is recommended.

Prognosis

Survival of children with differentiated thyroid cancer is excellent. Fortunately, it is very rare that a child dies of thyroid cancer. Childhood thyroid cancers are seldom undifferentiated. However, occasionally, a differentiated cancer that has not been excised or ablated transforms to anaplastic cancer and results in death. This occurred in 1 patient of 34 in a series from Hong Kong, 18 years after the primary treatment.[46] The majority of publications cited in this chapter do not document a single death. Buckwalter et al.[47] believe that one reason for the favorable outcome is that childhood cancers are more sensitive to TSH. However, the recurrence rate is significant and higher in those who present with cervical node metastases and in younger patients. A multivariate analysis of factors effecting outcome in 109 patients aged 6–17 years found that total thyroidectomy was the single most important factor for disease-free survival and was statistically significant.[48] [131]I improved disease-free survival but that did not reach statistical significance. An analysis of 327 children conducted by the Surgical Discipline Committee of the Children's

Cancer Group reported no death at 10 years.[6] The 5- and 10-year disease-free survivals were 76% and 66%, respectively. These reports highlight the need for long-term follow-up and the recognition that there can be setbacks but they should be addressed by diagnostic FNA, surgical excision of palpable cancers, and ^{131}I for nonpalpable recurrences. Even when a very poor outcome might be expected, for example, in a child presenting with extensive invasive cancer, cervical and distant metastases, the outcome can be favorable after treatment by total thyroidectomy and [131]I.[49]

Summary

Thyroid cancer is not common in children but when a thyroid nodule or enlarged cervical node is recognized it is important to proceed to FNA for a tissue diagnosis. A skilled thyroid surgeon should conduct a total thyroidectomy. In some cases, ^{131}I is advised to ablate residual thyroid and definitely in the case of functioning metastases. The importance of a sensitive easily available physician for long-term follow-up is stressed.

References

1. Wu Y. Differentiated carcinoma of the thyroid in children and adolescents. Ann Chir 2001;126(10):977–980.
2. Farahati J, Parlowsky T, Mader U, Reiners C, Bucsky P. Differentiated thyroid cancer in children and adolescents. Langenbecks Arch Surg 1998;383(3–4): 235–239.
3. De Keyser LF, Van Herle AJ. Differentiated thyroid cancer in children. Head Neck Surg 1985;8(2):100–114.
4. Nagai G, Pitts W, Basso L, Cisco JA, McDougall IR. Scintigraphic "hot nodules" and thyroid carcinoma. Clin Nucl Med 1987;12:123–127.
5. Corrias A, Einaudi S, Chiorboli E, et al. Accuracy of fine needle aspiration biopsy of thyroid nodules in detecting malignancy in childhood: comparison with conventional clinical, laboratory, and imaging approaches. J Clin Endocrinol Metab 2001;86:4484–4488.
6. La Quaglia MP, Black T, Holcomb GW 3rd, et al. Differentiated thyroid cancer: clinical characteristics, treatment, and outcome in patients under 21 years of age who present with distant metastases. A report from the Surgical Discipline Committee of the Children's Cancer Group. J Pediatr Surg 2000;35(6):955–959; discussion 960.
7. Peretz A, Leiberman E, Kapelushnik J, Hershkovitz E. Thyroglossal duct carcinoma in children: case presentation and review of the literature. Thyroid 2004;14(9): 777–785.

8. Nikiforov YE, Erickson LA, Nikiforova MN, Caudill CM, Lloyd RV. Solid variant of papillary thyroid carcinoma: incidence, clinical-pathologic characteristics, molecular analysis, and biologic behavior. Am J Surg Pathol 2001;25(12):1478–1484.

9. Hassoun AA, Hay ID, Goellner JR, Zimmerman D. Insular thyroid carcinoma in adolescents: a potentially lethal endocrine malignancy. Cancer 1997;79(5): 1044–1048.

10. Ringel M, Levine MA. Current therapy for childhood thyroid cancer: optimal surgery and the legacy of King Pyrrhus. Ann Surg Oncol 2002;10:4–6.

11. Bal CS, Padhy AK, Kumar A. Clinical features of differentiated thyroid carcinoma in children and adolescents from a sub-Himalayan iodine-deficient endemic zone. Nucl Med Commun 2001;22(8):881–887.

12. Arici C, Erdogan O, Altunbas H, et al. Differentiated thyroid carcinoma in children and adolescents. Clinical characteristics, treatment and outcome of 15 patients. Horm Res 2002;57(5–6):153–156.

13. Kowalski LP, Goncalves Filho J, Pinto CA, Carvalho AL, de Camargo B. Long-term survival rates in young patients with thyroid carcinoma. Arch Otolaryngol Head Neck Surg 2003;129(7):746–749.

14. Cady B. Presidential address: beyond risk groups—a new look at differentiated thyroid cancer. Surgery 1998;124(6):947–957.

15. Miccoli P, Antonelli A, Spinelli C, Ferdeghini M, Fallahi P, Baschieri L. Completion total thyroidectomy in children with thyroid cancer secondary to the Chernobyl accident. Arch Surg 1998;133(1):89–93.

16. Jarzab B, Handkiewicz-Junak D, Wloch J. Juvenile differentiated thyroid carcinoma and the role of radioiodine in its treatment: a qualitative review. Endocr Relat Cancer 2005;12(4):773–803.

17. Zimmerman D, Hay ID, Gough IR, et al. Papillary thyroid cancer in children and adults: long-term follow-up of 1039 patients conservatively treated at one institute during three decades. Surgery 1988;104:1157–1166.

18. Park H-M, Perkins OW, Edmondson JW, et al. Influence of diagnostic radioiodines on the uptake of ablative dose of iodine-131. Thyroid 1994;4:49–54.

19. McDougall IR. 74 MBq radioiodine 131I does not prevent uptake of therapeutic doses of 131I (i.e. it does not cause stunning) in differentiated thyroid cancer. Nucl Med Commun 1997;18(6):505–512.

20. Park HM. 123I: almost a designer radioiodine for thyroid scanning. J Nucl Med 2002;43(1):77–78.

21. Mandel SJ, Shankar LK, Benard F, Yamamoto A, Alavi A. Superiority of iodine-123 compared with iodine-131 scanning for thyroid remnants in patients with differentiated thyroid cancer. Clin Nucl Med 2001;26(1):6–9.

22. Mazzaferri EL. Radioiodine and other treatments and outcomes. In: Braverman LE, Utiger RD, eds. Werner and Inbar's The Thyroid: A Fundamental and Clinical Text. 8th ed. Philadelphia: Lippincott Williams & Wilkins; 2000:904–929.

23. Hung W, Sarlis NJ. Current controversies in the management of pediatric patients with well-differentiated nonmedullary thyroid cancer: a review. Thyroid 2002;12(8): 683–702.

24. Haveman JW, van Tol KM, Rouwe CW, Piers do A, Plukker JT. Surgical experience in children with differentiated thyroid carcinoma. Ann Surg Oncol 2003;10(1): 15–20.

25. Chow SM, Law SC, Mendenhall WM, et al. Differentiated thyroid carcinoma in childhood and adolescence: clinical course and role of radioiodine. Pediatr Blood Cancer 2004;42(2):176–183.

26. Grigsby PW, Gal-or A, Michalski JM, Doherty GM. Childhood and adolescent thyroid carcinoma. Cancer 2002;95(4):724–729.

27. Samuel AM, Rajashekharrao B, Shah DH. Pulmonary metastases in children and adolescents with well-differentiated thyroid cancer. J Nucl Med 1998;39(9): 1531–1536.

28. Anger K, Feine U. Thyroid carcinoma in childhood. Prog Pediatr Surg 1983;16: 39–42.

29. Schlumberger M. Papillary and follicular thyroid carcinoma. N Engl J Med 1998; 338:297–306.

30. Sisson JC, Carey JE. Thyroid carcinoma with high levels of function: treatment with (131)I. J Nucl Med 2001;42(6):975–883.

31. Sisson JC, Shulkin BL, Lawson S. Increasing efficacy and safety of treatments of patients with well-differentiated thyroid carcinoma by measuring body retentions of 131I. J Nucl Med 2003;44(6):898–903.

32. Haugen BR, Pacini F, Reiners C, et al. A comparison of recombinant human thyrotropin and thyroid hormone withdrawal for the detection of thyroid remnant or cancer. J Clin Endocrinol Metab 1999;84(11):3877–3885.

33. Iorcansky S, Herzovich V, Qualey RR, Tuttle RM. Serum thyrotropin (TSH) levels after recombinant human TSH injections in children and teenagers with papillary thyroid cancer. J Clin Endocrinol Metab 2005;90(12):6553–6555.

34. Grigsby PW, Siegel BA, Baker S, Eichling JO. Radiation exposure from outpatient radioactive iodine (131I) therapy for thyroid carcinoma. JAMA 2000;283(17): 2272–2274.

35. Sisson JC, Giordano TJ, Jamadar DA, et al. 131-I treatment of micronodular pulmonary metastases from papillary thyroid carcinoma. Cancer 1996;78(10):2184–2192.

36. Rosenbaum RC, Johnston GS, Valente WA. Frequency of hepatic visualization during I-131 imaging for metastatic thyroid carcinoma. Clin Nucl Med 1988;13(9): 657–660.

37. Carlisle M, Lu C, McDougall IR. The interpretation of 131I scans in the evaluation of thyroid cancer, with an emphasis on false positive findings. Nucl Med Commun 2003;24:715–735.

38. Vini L, Hyer S, Al-Saadi A, Pratt B, Harmer C. Prognosis for fertility and ovarian function after treatment with radioiodine for thyroid cancer. Postgrad Med J 2002;78(916):92–93.

39. Casara D. Rubello D, Saladini G, et al. Pregnancy after high therapeutic doses of iodine-131 in differentiated thyroid cancer: potential risks and recommendations. Eur J Nucl Med 1993;20(3):192–194.

40. Dottorini ME, Lomuscio G, Mazzucchelli L, Vignati A, Colombo L. Assessment of female fertility and carcinogenesis after iodine-131 therapy for differentiated thyroid carcinoma. J Nucl Med 1995;36(1):21–27.

41. Ayala C, Navarro E, Rodriguez JR, Silva H, Venegas E, Astorga R. Conception after iodine-131 therapy for differentiated thyroid cancer. Thyroid 1998;8(11):1009–1011.

42. Dottorini ME, Vignati A, Mazzucchelli L, Lomuscio G, Colombo L. Differentiated thyroid carcinoma in children and adolescents: a 37-year experience in 85 patients. J Nucl Med 1997;38(5):669–675.

43. Hyer S, Vini L, O'Connell M, Pratt B, Harmer C. Testicular dose and fertility in men following I(131) therapy for thyroid cancer. Clin Endocrinol (Oxf) 2002;56(6): 755–758.

44. Rall JE, Alpers JB, Lewallen CG, Sonenberg M, Berman M, Rawson RW. Radiation pneumonitis and fibrosis: a complication of radioiodine treatment of pulmonary metastases from cancer of the thyroid. J Clin Endocrinol Metab 1957;17(11): 1263–1276.

45. Alessandri AJ, Goddard KJ, Blair GK, Fryer CJ, Schultz KR. Age is the major determinant of recurrence in pediatric differentiated thyroid carcinoma. Med Pediatr Oncol 2000;35(1):41–46.

46. Lee YM, Lo CY, Lam KY, Wan KY, Tam PK. Well-differentiated thyroid carcinoma in Hong Kong Chinese patients under 21 years of age: a 35-year experience. J Am Coll Surg 2002;194(6):711–716.

47. Buckwalter JA, Thomas CG, Freeman JB. Is childhood thyroid cancer a lethal disease? Ann Surg 1975;181(5):632–639.

48. Jarzab B, Handkiewicz Junak D, Wloch J, et al. Multivariate analysis of prognostic factors for differentiated thyroid carcinoma in children. Eur J Nucl Med 2000;27(7):833–841.

49. Zettinig G, Kaserer K, Passler C, Flores JA, Niederle B, Dudczak R. Advanced insular thyroid carcinoma in a fourteen-year-old girl: twenty-four years of follow-up. Thyroid 2000;10(5):435–437.

8. Thyroid Cancer and Pregnancy

The majority of babies are born to young women. Thyroid cancer is a disease of young women. When thyroid cancer is diagnosed during pregnancy, the physician has to manage two patients.

Thyroid Nodule in Pregnancy

Two to five percent of normal young women have a thyroid nodule.[1] In nonpregnant women, approximately 5%–6% of nodules are cancerous.[2] Some authorities put the likelihood of cancer in the pregnant woman as high as 39%–43%.[3] In one study, the incidence of papillary cancer in pregnancy and puerperium was 21% and 3.4% in controls.[4] Overall, a risk of about 10% is more realistic. In a euthyroid patient, the optimal diagnostic procedure is a fine needle aspiration (FNA) of the nodule.[5] In a pregnant patient, there is debate whether it should be done during the pregnancy or after delivery of the baby. The arguments for waiting are that the risk of cancer is small, probably using the figure 10%, and papillary cancer grows slowly and has an excellent prognosis, plus the risk of operating during pregnancy. The opposite point of view is based on the higher likelihood of cancer and the risk of more rapid cancer growth with invasion and metastases.[6] Surgery in a pregnant woman is safe for mother and fetus and in most cases the patient and physician want to know the diagnosis and would proceed with FNA and when there is evidence of cancer deal with that surgically. However, when the nodule is found in the third trimester, it is reasonable to delay FNA until after delivery.

When the free hormones are increased and thyrotropin (TSH) is low, the patient has either an autonomous nodule or Graves' disease with a nonfunctioning nodule. In a nonpregnant patient, this would be resolved by scintiscan using ^{123}I but this test is contraindicated during pregnancy and FNA is advised.

An indeterminate FNA diagnosis is reported in 10%–20% of nodules and 80%–85% of these turn out to be benign. This is a therapeutic dilemma, but I wait until after delivery before referring for surgery. FNA showing a benign nodule should lead to periodic clinical follow-up examinations.

Treatment of Thyroid Cancer Diagnosed in Pregnancy

There is usually no reason to advise an abortion and the goal is to have a healthy mother and baby. The timing of surgery is determined by the stage of the pregnancy. Cancer diagnosed early in pregnancy can be removed safely in the second trimester.[7] After thyroidectomy, ^{131}I must not be administered to a pregnant or nursing woman. It is preferable to have a low-normal TSH rather than a suppressed one. The omission of ^{131}I treatment and a suppressed TSH for several months in a young woman with papillary cancer should have no adverse effect. In late pregnancy, surgery can be delayed about 3 months after delivery. Driggers et al.[8] reported on a woman diagnosed early in pregnancy by FNA to have papillary cancer. A decision was made to defer surgery until after the delivery. The lesion grew and at surgery the cancer was found to have invaded the trachea and recurrent laryngeal nerve and metastasized to lymph nodes. Therefore, when surgery is not advised, the patient needs to be followed by careful clinical examinations.

The surgery can be conducted under general anesthesia but local anesthetic has a role. Although this is not the common approach, several surgeons have published their results.[9,10] The surgeon should be experienced in thyroid operative procedures and have a low complication rate. Levothyroxine is started before surgery and the dose titrated to keep the TSH at the low level of normal. It is reasonable to start with 0.15 mg daily and check levels after 6 weeks and then titrate the dose dependent on TSH.[11–13] In pregnant women, total thyroid hormone values are usually increased and more reliance should be given to free thyroxine (FT_4) and TSH. Oral iron and calcium have a significant effect in reducing the absorption of L-thyroxine from the gastrointestinal tract, therefore prenatal vitamin and mineral preparations should be taken several hours apart from thyroid hormone.[14,15] The patient should have measurements of FT_4 and TSH at intervals of 6 weeks to ensure that she is euthyroid. I do not recommend measuring thyroglobulin (Tg) at this time because nothing is going to be done about the value until after delivery.

After delivery, the dose of L-thyroxine decreases and thyroid function tests are recommended at the 6-week postpartum follow-up.[13] Tg should be measured now. This value, along with the pathology results and surgical findings, are used to determine whether there should be testing and treatment with radioiodine. Because the patient is a young woman, she is usually in the best prognostic group. Most patients will be Stage I or low MACIS (metastasis, age, completeness of resection, invasion, and size) scores, thus predicting an excellent outcome. The patient with a small intrathyroidal cancer that has been totally excised would not benefit from [131]I. When the Tg is undetectable, the patient can be followed by clinical examination, measurement of thyroid function and Tg at intervals of 6 months over several years and then annually. Long-term follow-up of patients at the Mayo Clinic who had low MACIS scores demonstrated no benefit from [131]I.[16] There is a role for ^{131}I for large, invasive, incompletely excised cancers and those with nodal metastases. The implications of administering ^{131}I to a woman who has recently delivered a baby are substantial. The sodium iodide symporter is active in breast tissue.[17,18] The maternal breast and the baby would be exposed to radiation. No testing or treatment with any radionuclide of iodine should be considered while a patient is breast-feeding. The breast has been identified on whole-body scans (Figure 8.1).[19,20] Therefore, treatment with ^{131}I could expose the breast, which is a radiosensitive organ to a substantial dose of radiation and there is evidence of an increased incidence of breast cancer in women with a prior

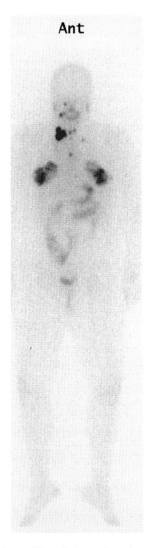

Figure 8.1. Uptake in the breasts bilaterally in a patient who was nursing up to the time of the scintiscan. This patient was not being managed at Stanford.

diagnosis of thyroid cancer.[21] I try to wait 6 months after the patient stops nursing before proceeding with diagnostic scanning with ^{123}I and therapy with [131]I. After treatment with ^{131}I, the mother is radioactive and has to be separated from her child.[22] The logistics need to be worked out well in advance.

TSH should be increased and the patient on a low iodine diet for 2 weeks. Serum Tg is measured and a negative pregnancy test needs to be documented. Whole-body scan is obtained 24 hours after 74–148 MBq (2–4 mCi) [123]I. The patient is then treated with a dose of ^{131}I based on the scan findings and stage of cancer. L-Thyroxine is started after 24 hours and the low iodine diet replaced by regular food at that time. A posttreatment scan is obtained after 6–8 days. The emitted radiation at this time determines whether the mother can be reunited with the baby. A follow-up visit is arranged for 6–8 weeks to confirm thyroid function is in the appropriate range aiming for a low or low normal TSH. Tg would also be measured to compare with the pretreatment value. When the thyroid tests are physiologic and the Tg value low, the patient is scheduled for a visit in 6 months.

There is debate whether differentiated cancer is more aggressive during pregnancy but we and others do not find that to be the case.[23,24] A study comparing the outcome in 61 pregnant women and 528 matched controls concluded the outcome was not statistically different.[6]

Management of Patient with Thyroid Cancer Who Wants to Become Pregnant

A young woman with treated thyroid cancer might desire to have a baby. When the patient has had a thyroidectomy, she can try to conceive after 6–8 weeks. This is to allow time to recover from the stress of the diagnosis and surgery and to ensure the dose of replacement L-thyroxine is appropriate and serum calcium is normal. The dose of L-thyroxine should be adjusted to maintain TSH at the low end of normal because suppressed TSH values can cause menstrual abnormalities and reduced fertility. It is recommended to wait about 12 months in a patient treated with [131]I. My philosophy is to have a follow-up scan and measurement of a stimulated Tg to ensure the therapy was successful. This would usually be conducted 6–12 months after ^{131}I treatment and a delay of 3 months after that is reasonable, hence a delay of 9–15 months.

Effect of ^{131}I on Fertility and Offspring

Women can conceive, carry a pregnancy, and have normal babies after they have been treated for thyroid cancer.[25–27] Direct measurements of radiation in the uterus indicate an absorbed dose of 0.18 rad/mCi (0.18 cGy/ 37 MBq).[28,29] This would not cause ovarian failure. Schlumberger et al.[25] noted an increased incidence of miscarriage in the year after ^{131}I probably related to abnormal thyroid function rather than gonadal radiation. There was no difference in the offspring after radioiodine treatment compared with those born before treatment. Vini et al.[27] found only one woman who wished to become pregnant could not. An increase in anomalies has been described in children conceived within a year of maternal ^{131}I.[30] This argues for a delay of 12 months that fits well with my philosophy.

Management of Pregnant Patient with Previously Treated Thyroid Cancer

When the patient is pregnant, the central issue is maintenance of the best health possible for mother and child. The patient should be advised to contact her physician as soon as pregnancy is suspected or confirmed. Referral to an obstetrician who will be responsible for monitoring the pregnancy and the delivery should be made. The requirement for L-thyroxine increases as the pregnancy advances.[12,31] Testing at 6-week intervals and readjustment of L-thyroxine are recommended through the entire 9 months. Supplemental iron, vitamins, minerals, and folic acid should be taken but iron and calcium should be taken several hours apart from the thyroid medication.[14,15] Children born to women who are hypothyroid throughout pregnancy can have a reduced IQ. In addition, hypothyroidism can result in maternal hypertension, preeclampsia, and premature delivery.[11,32]

Effects of Cancer on the Pregnancy and Pregnancy on the Cancer

The cancer should have no adverse effects on the pregnancy provided thyroid function is kept physiologic. There is no report of cancer spreading from patient to fetus. There is some evidence to suggest that thyroid cancer is more aggressive during pregnancy because of stimulation by human chorionic gonadotropin.[3,33] We and others found the natural history to be similar to thyroid cancer in nonpregnant women.[23,34]

Inadvertent Exposure of Pregnant Patient to Internal Radiation

The fetus should not be exposed to radiation and radioiodine, for testing or therapy is contraindicated during pregnancy. The fetal thyroid traps iodine at about the 10th–11th week. A relatively small dose of ^{131}I administered to the mother can ablate the fetal gland and cause permanent hypothyroidism. Authorities state clearly the patient should not be pregnant when treated but how this is to be practiced is less clear. The United Kingdom guidelines say, "No patient in whom there is a chance of being pregnant may receive radioiodine therapy; *if necessary* a pregnancy test should be performed."[35] Stoffer and Hamburger[36] polled 963 members of the American Thyroid Association and the Endocrine Society and obtained reports of 237 patients who were treated with ^{131}I when pregnant. Fifty-five patients were advised to have a therapeutic abortion and 182 were advised that it would be safe to continue with the pregnancy. Younger fetuses were at low risk of hypothyroidism and there was no increase in congenital abnormalities. The authors state, "We assumed by this time everyone administering ^{131}I therapy would routinely perform a pregnancy test," and "It is difficult to justify reliance upon menstrual history." Fisher et al.[37] presented the case of a mother who received 536.5 MBq (14.5 mCi) when the fetus was 3 months. The fetal thyroid absorbed about 250,000 rad (2500 Gy). Another patient underwent ^{131}I treatment with a dose of 500 MBq (13.5 mCi) and 10 days later was recognized to be 22 weeks pregnant.[38] The fetal thyroid absorbed 600 Gy (60,000 rad). Evans et al.[39] presented three women who were found to be pregnant at the time of ^{131}I treatment. The fetuses were 4–6 weeks, 7 weeks, and 8 weeks old when exposed to [131]I. No pregnancy tests were obtained. The doses ranged from 370 to 572 MBq (10–15.5 mCi) and none of the babies was hypothyroid. This illustrates the importance of fetal age and damage to thyroid from [131]I. When a fetus 10 weeks or older is exposed in utero it would be wise to start L-thyroxine immediately after delivery. The hope would be that normal physical and mental development would follow. There are reports of treatment with intraamniotic triiodothyronine and then L-thyroxine for a fetal goiter and hypothyroidism.[40] This should be under the management of an obstetrician skilled in the procedure. Exposure of the baby to 1 Gy (100 rad) results in a 3% risk of cancer and a reduction of 30 points in IQ. Documentation of a negative pregnancy test is important before administration of ^{131}I and the responsibility lies with the treating doctor. A recent court report illustrates that a signature of a technologist who verified the patient did not think she was pregnant was insufficient evidence.[41]

Summary and Key Facts

Thyroid nodules are identified in 2%–5% of pregnant women. The incidence of cancer in a nodule is greater in pregnancy. The best test is FNA. When thyroid cancer is diagnosed in early pregnancy, it can be removed safely by surgery in the second trimester. Patients who are pregnant or nursing should not receive diagnostic or therapeutic radioiodine. When a woman of childbearing age is treated with ^{131}I, it is important to document that there is no possibility of pregnancy.

References

1. Morris PC. Thyroid cancer complicating pregnancy. Obstet Gynecol Clin North Am 1998;25(2):401–405.

2. Gharib H. Fine-needle aspiration biopsy of thyroid nodules: advantages, limitations, and effect. Mayo Clin Proc 1994;69:44–49.

3. Rosen IB, Walfish PG. Pregnancy as a predisposing factor in thyroid neoplasia. Arch Surg 1986;121(11):1287–1290.

4. Marley EF, Oertel YC. Fine-needle aspiration of thyroid lesions in 57 pregnant and postpartum women. Diagn Cytopathol 1997;16(2):122–125.

5. Goldman MH, Tisch B, Chattock AG. Fine-needle biopsy of a solitary thyroid nodule arising during pregnancy. J Med Soc N J 1983;80(7):525–526.

6. Moosa M, Mazzaferri EL. Outcome of differentiated thyroid cancer diagnosed in pregnant women. J Clin Endocrinol Metab 1997;82(9):2862–2866.

7. Brodsky JB, Cohen EN, Brown BW Jr, Wu ML, Whitcher C. Surgery during pregnancy and fetal outcome. Am J Obstet Gynecol 1980;138(8):1165–1167.

8. Driggers RW, Kopelman JN, Satin AJ. Delaying surgery for thyroid cancer in pregnancy. A case report. J Reprod Med 1998;43(10):909–912.

9. Hochman M, Fee WE Jr. Thyroidectomy under local anesthesia. Arch Otolaryngol Head Neck Surg 1991;117(4):405–407.

10. Hisham AN, Aina EN. A reappraisal of thyroid surgery under local anaesthesia: back to the future? ANZ J Surg 2002;72(4):287–289.

11. Mandel SJ. Hypothyroidism and chronic autoimmune thyroiditis in the pregnant state: maternal aspects. Best Pract Res Clin Endocrinol Metab 2004;18(2):213–224.

12. McDougall IR, Maclin N. Hypothyroid women need more thyroxine when pregnant. J Fam Pract 1995;41(3):238–240.

13. Kaplan MM. Management of thyroxine therapy during pregnancy. Endocr Pract 1996;2(4):281–286.

14. Campbell NR, Hasinoff BB, Stalts H, Rao B, Wong NC. Ferrous sulfate reduces thyroxine efficacy in patients with hypothyroidism. Ann Intern Med 1992;117(12):1010–1013.

15. Shakir KM, Chute JP, Aprill BS, Lazarus AA. Ferrous sulfate-induced increase in requirement for thyroxine in a patient with primary hypothyroidism. South Med J 1997;90(6):637–639.

16. Hay ID, Thompson GB, Grant CS, et al. Papillary thyroid carcinoma managed at the Mayo Clinic during six decades (1940–1999): temporal trends in initial therapy and long-term outcome in 2444 consecutively treated patients. World J Surg 2002;26(8):879–885.

17. Wapnir IL, van de Rijn M, Nowels K, et al. Immunohistochemical profile of the sodium/iodide symporter in thyroid, breast, and other carcinomas using high density tissue microarrays and conventional sections. J Clin Endocrinol Metab 2003;88(4):1880–1888.

18. Dohan O, De la Vieja A, Paroder V, et al. The sodium/iodide symporter (NIS): characterization, regulation, and medical significance. Endocr Rev 2003;24(1):48–77.

19. Bakheet SM, Hammami MM. Patterns of radioiodine uptake by the lactating breast. Eur J Nucl Med 1994;21(7):604–608.

20. Bakheet SM, Powe J, Hammami MM. Unilateral radioiodine breast uptake. Clin Nucl Med 1998;23(3):170–171.

21. Chen AY, Levy L, Goepfert H, Brown BW, Spitz MR, Vassilopoulou-Sellin R. The development of breast carcinoma in women with thyroid carcinoma. Cancer 2001; 92(2):225–231.

22. Barrington SF, O'Doherty MJ, Kettle AG, et al. Radiation exposure of the families of outpatients treated with radioiodine (iodine-131) for hyperthyroidism. Eur J Nucl Med 1999;26(7):686–692.

23. Choe W, McDougall IR. Thyroid cancer in pregnant women: diagnostic and therapeutic management. Thyroid 1994;4(4):433–435.

24. Wemeau JL, Do CaoC. [Thyroid nodule, cancer and pregnancy]. Ann Endocrinol (Paris) 2002;63(5):438–442.

25. Schlumberger M, De Vathaire F, Ceccarelli C, et al. Exposure to radioactive iodine-131 for scintigraphy or therapy does not preclude pregnancy in thyroid cancer patients. J Nucl Med 1996;37(4):606–612.

26. Chow SM, Yau S, Lee SH, Leung WM, Law SC. Pregnancy outcome after diagnosis of differentiated thyroid carcinoma: no deleterious effect after radioactive iodine treatment. Int J Radiat Oncol Biol Phys 2004;59(4):992–1000.

27. Vini L, Hyer S, Al-Saadi A, Pratt B, Harmer C. Prognosis for fertility and ovarian function after treatment with radioiodine for thyroid cancer. Postgrad Med J 2002; 78(916):92–93.

28. Briere J, Philippon B. Absorbed dose to ovaries or uterus during a 131I-therapeutic of cancer or hyperthyroidism: comparison between in vivo measurements by TLD and calculations. Int J Appl Radiat Isot 1979;30(10):643–646.

29. Philippon B, Briere J. Absorbed dose to ovaries and uterus during 131I-treatment of hyperthyroidism: comparison between in vivo TLD measurements and calculations. Health Phys 1979;36(6):727–729.

30. Ayala C, Navarro E, Rodriguez JR, Silva H, Venegas E, Astorga R. Conception after iodine-131 therapy for differentiated thyroid cancer. Thyroid 1998;8(11):1009–1011.

31. Alexander EK, Marqusee E, Lawrence J, Jarolim P, Fischer GA, Larsen PR. Timing and magnitude of increases in levothyroxine requirements during pregnancy in women with hypothyroidism. N Engl J Med 2004;351(3):241–249.

32. Krassas GE. Thyroid disease and female reproduction. Fertil Steril 2000;74(6): 1063–1070.

33. Kobayashi K, Tanaka Y, Ishiguro S, Mori T. Rapidly growing thyroid carcinoma during pregnancy. J Surg Oncol 1994;55(1):61–64.

34. Vini L, Hyer S, Pratt B, Harmer C. Management of differentiated thyroid cancer diagnosed during pregnancy. Eur J Endocrinol 1999;140(5):404–406.

35. Lazarus JH. Guidelines for the use of radioiodine in the management of hyperthyroidism: a summary. Prepared by the Radioiodine Audit Subcommittee of the Royal College of Physicians Committee on Diabetes and Endocrinology, and the Research Unit of the Royal College of Physicians. J R Coll Physicians Lond 1995;29(6): 464–469.

36. Stoffer SS, Hamburger JI. Inadvertent 131I therapy for hyperthyroidism in the first trimester of pregnancy. J Nucl Med 1976;17(02):146–149.

37. Fisher WD, Voorhess ML, Gardner LI. Congenital hypothyroidism in infant following maternal I-131 therapy with a review of hazards of environmental radioisotope contamination. J Pediatr 1963;62:132–146.

38. Berg GE, Nystrom EH, Jacobsson L, et al. Radioiodine treatment of hyperthyroidism in a pregnant women. J Nucl Med 1998;39(2):357–361.

39. Evans PM, Webster J, Evans WD, Bevan JS, Scanlon MF. Radioiodine treatment in unsuspected pregnancy. Clin Endocrinol (Oxf) 1998;48(3):281–283.

40. Agrawal P, Ogilvy-Stuart A, Lees C. Intrauterine diagnosis and management of congenital goitrous hypothyroidism. Ultrasound Obstet Gynecol 2002;19(5):501–505.

41. Berlin L. Iodine-131 and the pregnant patient. AJR Am J Roentgenol 2001;176(4):869–871.

9. Anaplastic Carcinoma of the Thyroid

Of the 53,856 thyroid cancers from the National Cancer Data Base, 1.7% were anaplastic cancers.[1] The proportion of anaplastic cancers can be as high as 16%, especially in countries where the intake of iodine is low.[2] The patient is usually 60 years or older and women are more often involved. This is the most lethal solid cancer and the median survival is about 3–6 months.[3,4] The only hope of cure is very early detection and complete excision. This seldom happens.

Etiology

Anaplastic cancer can arise from preexisting differentiated thyroid cancer.[5] In a minority of cases, the cancer erupts from a longstanding, apparently benign goiter; however, an undiagnosed preexisting differentiated cancer might have been present.[6] External radiation or internal ^{131}I radiation for differentiated cancer has been blamed for anaplastic transformation. Nine of 67 patients treated at the Massachusetts General Hospital had received [131]I.[7] The probability of an anaplastic cancer being the result of ^{131}I is low and has been estimated at about 5%–10%. Molecular genetics of anaplastic cancer support a "2 hit" cause. In poorly differentiated cancers, there is a high incidence of mutations in the cancer suppressor *p53* gene. In a metaanalysis, mutations were identified in *p53* in more than half of 265 anaplastic cancers.[8]

Anaplastic cancers are more frequent in regions of iodine deficiency, which in turn causes endemic goiter and multinodular goiter. In regions where iodine supplementation has been instituted, there has been a statistically significant reduction in the number and proportion of anaplastic cancers.[9] There is no direct evidence for familial anaplastic cancer.

Pathology

The cells are large, bizarre, and are often multinucleated with hyperchromatic nuclei and they do not look or behave like follicular cells. Using modern techniques, so-called small cell anaplastic cancers are now usually classified as lymphoma, or medullary cancer.

Clinical Features

The patients are almost always older than 60 years and there is a about a twofold increase in women. There is a rapidly enlarging neck mass that occurs in almost all patients.[10] Dysphagia, dyspnea, and dysphonia are each found in about 30%–50% of patients and many patients have more than one of these major symptoms.[11] The duration of symptoms is usually 2–6 weeks. Lymph node metastases are present in 80% and distant metastases in about 50% at the time of presentation.[12] The patient has a rock-hard, fixed thyroid mass that is usually more than 5 cm in diameter. About 20%–30% of patients have neck pain. The cancer can metastasize to any organ. The most frequent sites of distant metastases are the lungs and skeleton and less commonly to the brain and meninges. There are cases of metastases to very unusual sites including the heart, tonsil, adrenal, and small bowel. An erysipelas-like reaction can be the result of skin metastases.[13] Neutrophilia, leukemoid reaction, and pyrexia of unknown origin (or fever of unknown origin) have been described. Release of thyroid hormones resulting in symptoms and signs of thyrotoxicosis is rare. [14] This presentation is similar to subacute thyroiditis and has been called carcinomatous pseudothyroiditis.

Diagnosis

An early tissue diagnosis is important and this is achieved by immediate fine needle aspiration (FNA). Computed tomography (CT) scan helps define encroachment on the aerodigestive tract and blood vessels and whether there are pulmonary metastases. The differential diagnosis includes lymphoma of the thyroid, De Quervain's (subacute) thyroiditis, Reidel's thyroiditis, and rapidly growing but differentiated thyroid cancers including medullary and Hürthle cell cancer. FNA establishes the correct diagnosis. Most patients have normal thyroid function but as described above thyrotoxicosis can occur occasionally.[14]

[18]Fluorodeoxyglucose (FDG)–positron emission tomography (PET) or PET/computed tomography (CT) scan is helpful in selected patients to define the extent of disease (Figure 9.1). The uptake of [18]FDG is very intense in anaplastic cancers (high standardized uptake value) with the poorest differentiation. Thus, [18]FDG-PET defines the extent of local disease and metastases and the likely degree of aggressiveness of the cancer. Combined [18]FDG-PET/CT also provides anatomy. There is no role for scintigraphy with radionuclides of iodine.

Treatment

A team approach including a thyroidologist, pathologist, surgeon, radiation oncologist, and medical oncologist or rapid referral to an institute that can provide a team approach is recommended. There must be adequate relief

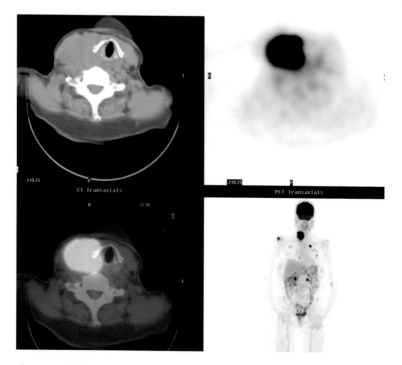

Figure 9.1. PET/CT scan 1 hour after injection of ^{18}FDG. The patient was an elderly woman with a long-standing goiter who noticed a change in its size. She had an FNA showing anaplastic thyroid cancer and was being evaluated for thyroidectomy. The scan shows a huge invasive primary cancer and widespread metastases proving that operation would be of no value.

of suffering with strong analgesia and sedatives. Treatments are surgery, external radiation, and chemotherapy. When the condition of the patient is satisfactory, combined therapy is recommended but there is no ideal multimodality protocol that is clearly superior and fits all. No matter how the patient is treated, the outcome is dismal.

Surgery

The only hope of long-term survival is when the cancer can be completely excised. This is usually only possible for anaplastic changes within a well-differentiated cancer. The mean survival in three patients with disease confined to the thyroid was 5.4 years, compared with 4.8 months in 81 patients with more advanced disease.[15] Treatment is designed to relieve local invasive symptoms as well as to improve survival. The prognosis is improved slightly by removal of the thyroid or debulking the cancer.[7,16] Complications from the surgery are more common because the cancer is invasive into surrounding structures.[7] Respiratory distress necessitates a tracheostomy. In patients with invasive disease, radical surgery does not improve the outcome compared with a less-invasive procedure.[17] However, thyroidectomy might be possible after combined chemotherapy and external radiation, provided the cancer shrinks. With regard to the thyroid operation, Clark[18] recommends removal of the more normal lobe first to identify anatomic landmarks such as the trachea. He emphasizes that because the surgery is palliative, every effort should be made to avoid complications.

External Radiation

External radiation is advised as the primary treatment when thyroidectomy is technically impossible. High-dose, external radiation should be administered to all patients should they live long enough. Some recommend this before operation and those who operate first support postoperative radiation. Hyperfractionation improves the survival slightly but there are complications including dry mouth, tracheitis, and esophagitis. Radiation osteonecrosis of the mandible has been described. Care must be taken to ensure that the spinal cord does not receive an excessive dose because, in one report, two patients died as a result of spinal cord necrosis.[19]

Chemotherapy

Adriamycin was originally shown by Kim and Leeper[20,21] to have benefit and is used in many chemotherapy combinations. A combination of adriamycin and cisplatinum resulted in three complete and three partial responses in 18 patients in contrast to one partial response to doxorubicin alone. Another report supported the combination of bleomycin, adriamycin, and cisplatinum.[22] Adriamycin is also a radiosensitizer. It is given in a dose of $10 \, mg/m^2$/wk (some use $20 \, mg/wk$). Even after original regression, the cancer usually recurs. Occasionally, chemotherapy causes sufficient reduction in size of the primary lesion to make it possible to consider surgical excision.

A multicenter trial using a 96-hour infusion of paclitaxel ($140 \, mg/m^2$) every 3 weeks was conducted on 19 patients.[23] One patient had a complete response and 7 (47%) had partial responses. The median survival in the responders was 32 weeks compared with 10 weeks in the nonresponders.

Multimodality Treatment

Multimodality treatment includes chemotherapy plus simultaneous radiation, e.g., 20 mg adriamycin weekly plus twice-daily external radiation of 1.6 Gy to a total of 46–60 Gy (4600–6000 rad). This can produce sufficient shrinkage of the cancer to allow thyroid debulking. Kim and Leeper[20] produced complete remission in 8 of 9 patients treated with adriamycin 10 mg/m^2 and hyperfractionated radiation of 160 cGy twice daily to a total of 57.6 Gy (5760 rad). In a separate investigation, 13 patients treated by surgery, external radiation, and chemotherapy had a significantly better outcome than 12 treated without operation or 8 who did not receive chemotherapy.[24] In this study, 21 patients who had local invasion of the cancer were excluded from the analysis and unfortunately many patients present in that way. In a report from the Mayo Clinic, multimodality treatment could not be demonstrated to improve the outcome.[12] These investigators reemphasized the "grim" prognosis and found that external radiation was somewhat beneficial in that the median survival was 5 months rather than 3 months. In contrast, investigators in San Francisco found a "reasonable prognosis" in patients treated by operation and then radiation and chemotherapy.[16] Results in 79 patients treated in Ljubljana found a better outcome when radiation and chemotherapy were delivered first (neoadjuvant therapy) and then the cancer was removed by operation.[25]

Brain metastases might be amenable to surgical excision if they are in a noncritical region. Otherwise, treatment by external radiation therapy or "gamma knife" should be prescribed.

In summary, multimodality treatment is recommended for anaplastic cancer of the thyroid. Small cancers that can be removed with minimal complication should be treated by operation followed by external radiation and chemotherapy. For large, invasive cancer, external radiation and chemotherapy are administered first and if the cancer shrinks surgery can be planned later. Veness et al.[26] summed up the situation: "Most patients with anaplastic thyroid cancer are incurable; however, a multimodality approach incorporating surgery and radiotherapy and chemotherapy, in selected individuals, might improve local control and extend survival."

Radioiodine

Anaplastic cancers do not express sodium iodide symporter. Therefore, in most patients, there is no role for ^{131}I. However, when there is dedifferentiation in the center of a differentiated cancer, it is advisable to ablate all functioning tissue with ^{131}I using the protocol described in Chapter 5. Reports of anaplastic cancers that show uptake of ^{131}I usually are explained by this relationship.[27] Retinoic acid has been administered with the intention and hope of increasing ^{131}I uptake by poorly differentiated cancers.[28] This is almost never successful for anaplastic cancer. Several weeks of pretreatment are necessary for retinoic acid, by which time the patient is usually dead.

Summary of Therapy

It seems that no matter how this cancer is treated, the outcome is extremely bad. There is some evidence that by combining surgery, radiation, and chemotherapy the survival is extended. Some favor operation first, others recommend the surgery should come after radiation and chemotherapy.

Prognosis

Anaplastic cancer has a dismal prognosis. Local disease is advanced and regional and or distant metastases are common at presentation. Patients with incidental anaplastic cancer should be analyzed separately from those with definitive anaplastic cancer. Few patients with nonincidental anaplastic thyroid cancer survive 1 year and most are dead in 3–6 months. In one report, 82% of the patients died within 1 year.[29] The median survival in another series of 91 patients was 21 weeks.[30] Despite the intensive treatment, 34 of 37 patients in a third series died within 1 year.[31] In a metaanalysis, the 2-year survival in 420 patients was 2.6%.[32] Rapid growth of the cancer, size >7 cm, dyspnea, dysphagia, old age, and distant metastases are poor prognostic indicators.[33]

Prophylaxis

The incidence of anaplastic cancer is decreasing probably because of earlier diagnosis and more effective therapy of papillary cancer. Correcting iodine deficiency by iodized salt is also a factor.

Summary and Key Points

Anaplastic cancer accounts for about 2% of thyroid cancers in regions of plentiful dietary iodine. It is the most aggressive solid cancer and few patients survive 6 months from diagnosis. The patients are elderly and might have a preexisting differentiated cancer or nodular goiter. The cancer grows very rapidly and causes local pressure effects and by the time of diagnosis there are nodal and distant metastases in 50%. Combination therapy with external radiation, systemic chemotherapy, and surgery produce a minimally better outcome.

References

1. Hundahl SA, Fleming ID, Fremgen AM, Menck HR. A National Cancer Data Base report on 53,856 cases of thyroid carcinoma treated in the U.S., 1985–1995 [see comments]. Cancer 1998;83(12):2638–2648.
2. Wenisch HJW, Wagner RH, Schumm-Draeger PM, Encke A. Cytostatic drug therapy in anaplastic thyroid carcinoma. World J Surg 1986;10(5):762–769.
3. Ain KB. Anaplastic thyroid carcinoma: a therapeutic challenge. Semin Surg Oncol 1999;16(1):64–69.
4. Pasieka JL. Anaplastic thyroid cancer. Curr Opin Oncol 2003;15(1):78–83.
5. Crile G Jr, Wilson DH. Transformation of a low grade papillary carcinoma of the thyroid to an anaplastic carcinoma after treatment with radioiodine. Surg Gynecol Obstet 1959;108(3):357–360.
6. Vescini F, Di Gaetano P, Vigna E, Pascoli A, Cacciari M. Anaplastic thyroid carcinoma in a 49-year-old woman with a long-standing goiter. A case report. Minerva Endocrinol 2000;25(3–4):81–83.
7. Pierie JP, Muzikansky A, Gaz RD, Faquin WC, Ott MJ. The effect of surgery and radiotherapy on outcome of anaplastic thyroid carcinoma. Ann Surg Oncol 2002; 9(1):57–64.
8. Lam KY, Lo CY, Chan KW, Wan KY. Insular and anaplastic carcinoma of the thyroid: a 45-year comparative study at a single institution and a review of the significance of p53 and p21. Ann Surg 2000;231(3):329–338.
9. Ratnatunga PC, Amarasinghe SC, Ratnatunga NV. Changing patterns of thyroid cancer in Sri Lanka. Has the iodination programme helped? Ceylon Med J 2003; 48(4):125–128.
10. Lo CY, Lam KY, Wan KY. Anaplastic carcinoma of the thyroid. Am J Surg 1999; 177(4):337–339.
11. Heron DE, Karimpour S, Grigsby PW. Anaplastic thyroid carcinoma: comparison of conventional radiotherapy and hyperfractionation chemoradiotherapy in two groups. Am J Clin Oncol 2002;25(5):442–446.
12. McIver B, Hay ID, Giuffrida DF, et al. Anaplastic thyroid carcinoma: a 50-year experience at a single institution. Surgery 2001;130(6):1028–1034.
13. Lee SY, Chang SE, Bae GY, et al. Carcinoma erysipeloides associated with anaplastic thyroid carcinoma. Clin Exp Dermatol 2001;26(8):671–673.
14. Villa ML, Mukherjee JJ, Tran NQ, Cheah WK, Howe HS, Lee KO. Anaplastic thyroid carcinoma with destructive thyrotoxicosis in a patient with preexisting multinodular goiter. Thyroid 2004;14(3):227–230.
15. Aldinger KA, Samaan NA, Ibanez M, Hill CS Jr. Anaplastic carcinoma of the thyroid: a review of 84 cases of spindle and giant cell carcinoma of the thyroid. Cancer 1978;41(6):2267–2275.
16. Haigh PI, Ituarte PH, Wu HS, et al. Completely resected anaplastic thyroid carcinoma combined with adjuvant chemotherapy and irradiation is associated with prolonged survival. Cancer 2001;91(12):2335–2342.

17. Venkatesh YS, Ordonez NG, Schultz PN, Hickey RC, Goepfert H, Samaan NA. Anaplastic carcinoma of the thyroid. A clinicopathologic study of 121 cases. Cancer 1990;66(2):321–330.

18. Kebebew E, Greenspan FS, Clark OH, Woeber KA, McMillan A. Anaplastic thyroid carcinoma. Treatment outcome and prognostic factors. Cancer 2005;103(7):1330–1335.

19. Simpson WJ. Anaplastic thyroid carcinoma: a new approach. Can J Surg 1980;23(1):25–27.

20. Kim JH, Leeper RD. Treatment of anaplastic giant and spindle cell carcinoma of the thyroid gland with combination adriamycin and radiation therapy. A new approach. Cancer 1983;52(6):954–957.

21. Kim JH, Leeper RD. Treatment of locally advanced thyroid carcinoma with combination doxorubicin and radiation therapy. Cancer 1987;60(10):2372–2375.

22. De Besi P, Busnardo B, Toso S, et al. Combined chemotherapy with bleomycin, adriamycin, and platinum in advanced thyroid cancer. J Endocrinol Invest 1991; 14(6):475–480.

23. Ain KB, Egorin MJ, DeSimone PA. Treatment of anaplastic thyroid carcinoma with paclitaxel: phase 2 trial using ninety-six-hour infusion. Collaborative Anaplastic Thyroid Cancer Health Intervention Trials (CATCHIT) Group. Thyroid 2000;10(7): 587–594.

24. Kasai N, Sakamoto A, Uchida M. A combined modality for anaplastic large-cell carcinoma of the thyroid. Auris Nasus Larynx 1985;12(suppl 2):S72–74.

25. Besic N, Auersperg M, Us-Krasovec M, Golouh R, Frkovic-Grazio S, Vodnik A. Effect of primary treatment on survival in anaplastic thyroid carcinoma. Eur J Surg Oncol 2001;27(3):260–264.

26. Veness MJ, Porter GS, Morgan GJ. Anaplastic thyroid carcinoma: dismal outcome despite current treatment approach. ANZ J Surg 2004;74(7):559–562.

27. Donovan JK, Ilbery PL. Metastases from anaplastic thyroid carcinoma responding to radioiodine. Clin Radiol 1971;22(3):401–404.

28. Schmutzler C, Kohrle J. Retinoic acid redifferentiation therapy for thyroid cancer. Thyroid 2000;10(5):393–406.

29. Carcangiu ML, Steeper T, Zampi G, Rosai J. Anaplastic thyroid carcinoma. A study of 70 cases. Am J Clin Pathol 1985;83(2):135–158.

30. Junor EJ, Paul J, Reed NS. Anaplastic thyroid carcinoma: 91 patients treated by surgery and radiotherapy. Eur J Surg Oncol 1992;18(2):83–88.

31. Kobayashi T, Asakawa H, Umeshita K, et al. Treatment of 37 patients with anaplastic carcinoma of the thyroid. Head Neck 1996;18(1):36–41.

32. Casterline PF, Jaques DA, Blom H, Wartofsky L. Anaplastic giant and spindle-cell carcinoma of the thyroid: a different therapeutic approach. Cancer 1980;45(7): 1689–1692.

33. Kihara M, Miyauchi A, Yamauchi A, Yokomise H. Prognostic factors of anaplastic thyroid carcinoma. Surg Today 2004;34(5):394–398.

10. Medullary Cancer

Medullary cancer arises from parafollicular cells (C cells) and account for 2%–5% of thyroid cancers. Seventy-five percent of patients have sporadic medullary cancer and 25% have familial medullary cancers that are transmitted as autosomal dominant and fall into three categories: 1) familial medullary cancers; 2) medullary cancer, pheochromocytoma, and or hyperparathyroidism, called multiple endocrine neoplasia 2A (MEN 2A); and 3) similar to 2A plus a characteristic phenotype described as marfanoid and neuromas of the lips, tongue, and intestine.

Etiology

Familial cases of medullary cancers are associated with a mutation in the *RET* protooncogene (Table 10.1).[1,2] *RET* has an extracellular domain that binds ligands and an adjacent region close to the cell membrane that is rich in cysteine molecules. The intracellular component contains the enzyme tyrosine kinase. The enzyme is activated when two *RET* molecules form a dimer and this occurs in the presence of an activating ligand. In medullary cancer, a base exchange in the gene results in substitution of an amino acid frequently replacing a cysteine. Cysteine molecules form intramolecular disulfide bridges but loss of a cysteine allows an unbridged molecule to combine with a free cysteine in a second monomer thus forming the dimer that activates intracellular tyrosine kinase. A missense mutation in any one of four codons in exon 10, two in exon 11, three in exon 13, and single defects in exon 14 predispose to MEN 2A (Figure 10.1). In MEN 2B, there have been two *RET* mutations identified in codon 16 and one in exon 15. In the case of familial medullary cancer not associated with MEN 2 syndromes, several of the same mutations found in MEN 2A have been identified. Genetic studies can identify individuals at risk for developing these syndromes and predict the phenotypic behavior of the cancer. A mutation in codon 634 of exon 11 accounts for more than half of the defects. Mutations in exons 13–16 cause intracellular missense mutations in the regions encoding the tyrosine kinase. These result in activation of the enzyme without the formation of a dimer.

Pathology

C cells are rare in normal thyroid and at high magnification can be seen to contain neurosecretory granules containing calcitonin. The cells stain positively with antibodies against calcitonin.[3] Approximately 80% of medullary

Table 10.1. Mutations associated with familial medullary cancer syndromes

Syndrome	Exon	Codon	Percentage with proven *RET* mutation
Familial medullary cancer	10	609, 611, 618, 620	85
	11	630, 634	
	13	768, 790, 791	
	14	804	
	15	891	
MEN 2A	10	609, 611, 618, 620	97
	11	630, 634	
	13	768	
MEN 2B	15	883	95
	16	918, 922	

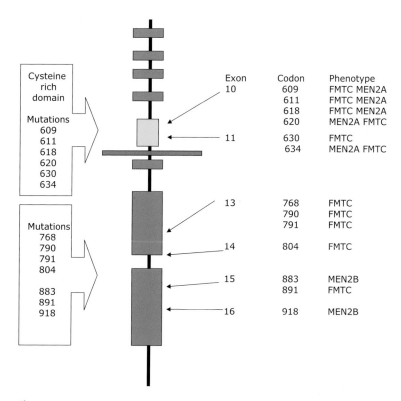

Figure 10.1. Diagrammatic representation of the *RET* protooncogene. It shows the position of amino acid substitutions resulting from mutations in the gene. The extramembranous site, the cysteine-rich site, and tyrosine kinase site are shown. (Adapted from McDougall IR. Management of Thyroid Cancer and Related Nodular Disease. London: Springer-Verlag; 2006:339.)

cancers contain amyloid. In hereditary syndromes there is a transition from normal to C cell hyperplasia and then to frank malignancy. Familial cancers can be bilateral and multifocal. Sporadic medullary cancer is usually a solitary lesion. Invasion of lymphatics, blood vessels, and surrounding soft tissues is common. Metastases to regional lymph nodes occur early.

Clinical Features

The most common presentation is an adult patient with no family history of medullary cancer who is found to have a thyroid nodule. About 10%–20% have local symptoms of dysphagia, dyspnea, or dysphonia.[4] The average age is 40–50 years and there is a very slight increase in women (1.1–1.5:1). The cytopathology from fine needle aspiration (FNA) indicates the diagnosis of medullary cancer. The cells stain for calcitonin and not thyroglobulin, confirming the diagnosis. The family history should be reviewed and genetic testing undertaken to define whether this is familial. When a germline mutation is present, family members should be investigated for this defect. Four families with seven patients were identified by screening 39 families in which the index patient was thought to have sporadic medullary thyroid cancer.[5] If the cancer is advanced and the patient has extensive metastatic disease, there can be troublesome watery diarrhea as a result of products secreted by the cancer.

The second presentation is when there is no FNA or when the FNA is indeterminate and the patient is referred to surgery to treat a thyroid nodule. The diagnosis is established after, rather than before, the operation. The difference is that appropriate investigations that are important before surgery have not been obtained and the surgical procedure is usually inadequate.

The final situation is identification of the patient by genetic screening because a relative has an established diagnosis. In MEN 2A and 2B, it is important to test for pheochromocytoma before conducting the thyroidectomy, because intraoperative hypertensive crisis can be avoided. Hyperparathyroidism produces hypercalcemia, which in turn can cause general malaise, tiredness, depression, dehydration, renal stones, and constipation. Cutaneous lichen amyloidosis is found in patients with MEN 2A. This is an itchy, papular rash of the skin in the back between C4 and T5 dermatomes. The patient with MEN 2B has a typical phenotype with long, thin arms, pectus abnormality of the chest, and neuromas of the lips and tongue. There are also intestinal neuromas that are not apparent clinically.

Diagnosis and Genetic Testing

The diagnosis of medullary cancer in a patient with a thyroid nodule is best achieved by FNA. Once the diagnosis has been established, it is important to conduct investigations to determine if the disease is familial, to stage the cancer, and to determine whether there are associated pathologies. Screening for *RET* protooncogene mutations located on exons 10, 11, 13–16 can be identified in peripheral white blood cells. When there is a *RET* mutation, the patient has familial thyroid cancer and with specific mutations there is a risk of pheochromocytoma or hyperparathyroidism. Absence of a mutation defines the patient does not have familial variety.

To rule in or out the diagnosis of pheochromocytoma, serum measurements of norepinephrine, epinephrine, and 24-hour urine measurements of these plus metanephrines and vinyl mandelic acid are obtained. When one of these investigations is abnormal, an anatomic image such as computed tomography (CT) or magnetic resonance imaging (MRI) should be obtained to determine the site or sites of the tumor. Treatment of pheochromocytoma takes precedence and should be undertaken by a surgical and anesthetic team experienced with this disorder. When serum calcium is high, a paired ionized calcium and parathormone level should be obtained. The diagnosis of hyperparathyroidism would result in a change in the thyroid operation. The abnormal parathyroid gland(s) would be removed during the total thyroidectomy.

Ultrasound and or CT of the neck is required to define the anatomy of the thyroid and determine whether there is more than one lesion, to examine central and lateral nodes for characteristics of metastatic disease, and to look for parathyroid abnormalities. Calcitonin and carcinoembryonic antigen (CEA) are measured and used for comparison during follow-up. When that calcitonin level is very elevated, there is increasing concern of regional and distant metastases. Distant lesions can occur in the liver, skeleton, and lungs. Liver metastases can be present early in the course of the disease. Occasionally, metastases to rare sites such as the breast and skin occur.[6–8] A positron emission tomography (PET) scan is excellent in identifying sizable metastases (>5–6 mm) but is not useful for miliary pulmonary or hepatic lesions. Helical CT of the chest and liver with thin sections after intravenous contrast should be conducted.

In all familial cancers, a team that looks after many patients with these diseases with combined skills in counseling, treatment, follow-up, and information for planning of pregnancy is advantageous. There has to be a discussion of the specific defect and what likelihood there is to develop medullary cancer (>95%), pheochromocytoma (approximately 50% for MEN 2A and 2B), and hyperparathyroidism (approximately 20%–30% for MEN 2A). Information about prognosis based on the type of syndrome and extent of disease should be presented. The probability that children are carriers and the need for screening relatives and the probability of finding disease should be presented. Negative aspects of genetic testing should also be addressed. Because the implications of having or not having a specific mutation are great and because no test is 100% sensitive and specific, some advise a duplicate genetic test especially when the test is negative and the family history is strong.[9] There needs to be great efforts to protect privacy. The emotional stress to gene carriers in particular children must be considered and follow-up should be arranged and where necessary referral for psychologic and or psychiatric consultation.

Measurement of calcitonin is accepted as a very valuable test to follow patients after operation. It is important to recognize that the sensitivity of different assays and the normal ranges vary considerably. In the past, basal and stimulated calcitonin values have been recommended to identify patients at risk for medullary cancer in kindreds who have one or other familial syndromes.[10–12] The use of these tests for screening families has been replaced by genetic testing. Measurement of calcitonin does have a role in follow-up of treated patients. Some authorities recommend measurement of calcitonin in patients with a thyroid nodule. Pacini et al. in 1994, and in an updated report, screened 10,864 patients with thyroid nodules and nodular goiter.[13] Forty-four patients (0.4%) with medullary cancer were identified. The cost of identifying a patient with medullary cancer was $12,500. However, FNA was suspicious for medullary cancer or thyroid cancer in 29 of the 44 (66%); 7276 consecutive patients with thyroid problems had calcitonin measurements.[14] Sixty-six patients had thyroidectomy, 45 (0.6% of the total group) had medullary cancer, and 16 (0.2%) had pathologic evidence of C cell hyperplasia. My judgment is that this screening is not cost-effective and FNA will identify most of the patients with isolated medullary cancer.

Hypercalcitonemia can occur in patients with chronic lymphocytic thyroiditis, pregnancy, chronic hypercalcemia, and those on hemodialysis.[15,16] An increased calcitonin was found in 4 of 161 hyperthyroid patients.[17] Measurement of calcitonin in a patient with a thyroid nodule is not recommended in the American Thyroid Association guidelines.[18]

Features of Cushing's syndrome including moon facies, striae, hypertension, and diabetes might be present in the rare patient whose cancer secretes adrenocorticotropic hormone (ACTH).[19–21]

Treatment

The treatment is based on the clinical presentation. There are published guidelines.[22,23] When the diagnosis is established by genetic testing, the main issue is whether there is evidence of pheochromocytoma or hyperparathyroidism. The mutation in *RET* protooncogene can help predict the patients most at risk for these. When there is a pheochromocytoma, it has to be treated first because untreated hypertensive crisis can occur during stressful situations such as thyroidectomy and cause death. Once that has been excluded or treated, patients with *RET* mutation who belong to families with MEN 2A should undergo total thyroidectomy by 5 years of age. Some authorities recommend an earlier operation for children with a defect in codon 634. In contrast, mutations in codons 609, 768, 790, 791, 804, and 891 have been associated with a more benign course and a better prognosis, and annual measurement of a stimulated calcitonin can be used to define the timing of surgery.[23,24] The goal is to remove the gland before there is clinical cancer. Often, C cell hyperplasia, which is the precursor of cancer, is diagnosed pathologically. Of

17 patients who underwent prophylactic operation at the M.D. Anderson Cancer Center, 12 had C cell hyperplasia but five had invasive disease.[25] None of the 17 patients died or had a recurrence. Similarly, 71 patients with a range of age from 10 months to 20 years underwent prophylactic thyroidectomy; 75% had abnormal basal calcitonin values and 68 of 71 had increased values after injection of pentagastrin.[26] Eighty-six percent (61 of 71) had medullary cancer and this was bilateral in 67% and >1 cm in 10%. This confirms the poor value of basal calcitonin for determining the best age for surgery. A recent report analyzed the pathologic findings in 207 patients diagnosed by genetic testing and operated on by the 20th year.[27] The patients came from 145 families of which the phenotypes were 112 with MEN 2A, 29 with familial medullary thyroid cancer, and four with MEN 2B. Development of both C cell hyperplasia and medullary cancer occurred earlier in families with mutations in the extracellular component of *RET*. In the case of extracellular defects, the average age for C cell hyperplasia was 8.3 years and for frank cancer 10.2 years. The corresponding ages for those with intracellular mutations were 11.2 and 16.6 years, respectively. Metastases to nodes were found at an average age of 17.1 years when the mutation was extracellular and none of eight patients with intracellular defects had metastases at age 20 years. Extracellular mutations were much more likely and affected 172 patients versus 31 with intracellular defects. Seven patients had nodal disease strengthening the decision for thyroidectomy at an early age. In patients with the most common mutation at codon 634, there was an average of 6.6 years between development of the cancer and the occurrence of metastases. The data suggest that surgery could be delayed to age 10 for those with mutations in codons 609, 630, 768, 790, 791, 804, and 891. Data such as this, if confirmed by other investigators, could allow more precise timing of operations for the individual patient. Because the onset of cancer and its metastases occur earlier in patients with MEN 2B, total thyroidectomy is recommended before the first birthday.[23]

There is disagreement about the need for central node dissection when surgery is conducted in young children. When there is no cancer in the thyroid, there is no chance of nodal metastases. Therefore, efforts should be made preoperatively to try to predict whether cancer has developed. An increased basal or calcium-stimulated calcitonin would be indications for nodal dissection. Also, when ultrasound demonstrates a mass in the thyroid or lymph nodes that have suspicious characteristics, the decision should be for thyroidectomy and central lymph node dissection. A cancer >1 cm and the presence of metastases to the central nodes would be an indication for excision of nodes from level II–VI. Because of the more aggressive behavior of medullary cancer in the MEN 2B syndrome, the recommendation for lymphadenectomy is based on a cancer size of >0.5 cm.

Operative complications in young children are problematic because they will persist for the life of the individual. Excised parathyroids can be autotransplanted. Total thyroidectomy and removal of the central neck nodes to level VI is the correct operation for those with established cancer. A proportion of patients with sporadic medullary cancer present with extensive local disease. It can be necessary to conduct extensive surgery.[28]

The Role of Postoperative Radiation and Chemotherapy

It was hoped that ^{131}I would have a role after surgery for medullary cancer by killing residual C cells that had the potential to become malignant and cause recurrences. This treatment has proven to be ineffective.[29] In one study, 15 patients were treated by operation and ^{131}I and compared with 84 treated by surgery. There was no difference in postoperative calcitonin values or 5- and 10-year survivals.

Treatment of distant metastases is a difficult problem. The cancer is relatively resistant to radiation and to chemotherapy.[30] Surgical debulking of large metastases has been shown to prolong survival.[31] This seems preferable to radiation therapy of mass lesions although radiation can help when smaller volumes of cancer are present after surgery.[32,33] Tubiana et al.[34] and Sarrazin et al.[35] showed that the outcome was equivalent in 80 patients who were treated by operation and 35 who had radiotherapy after surgery; nonetheless, they thought that radiation was helpful. This was because the irradiated patients had more advanced disease. Distant metastases were excluded as far as possible. Radiation has a role when there is residual cancer in the neck that cannot be removed by operation. It can also be used in patients with proven metastases to lymph nodes and persistently increased calcitonin values. It has a definitive place in treating painful skeletal metastases. Investigations to help find sites of cancer are discussed below. These results stress the goal of early diagnosis and definitive surgical treatment before nodal and distant lesions have developed.

Unsealed radiation therapy has been undertaken by a few investigators. The therapeutic potential of this should be tested by preliminary diagnostic imaging. ^{123}I-metaiodobenzylguanidine (MIBG) whole-body scan can be used as a preliminary to ^{131}I-MIBG treatment. MIBG labeled with ^{131}I has been investigated by several groups.[36,37] Its role in treatment of metastatic pheochromocytoma is more established than its use for medullary cancer.[38,39] [131]I monoclonal antibodies to CEA were infused into 12 patients with medullary cancer.[40] The dose was designed to cause myeloablation and the patients received autologous bone marrow transplantation about 2 weeks later. Radiolabeled octreotide has been prescribed to treat endocrine cancers including medullary cancer. Some investigators have used indium-111 (^{111}In)-octreotide. The Auger electrons from ^{111}In deliver a high dose over a very short path-length. Experimental studies have shown a ratio of uptake in the cancer compared with blood of 160:1, suggesting the treatment should be effective.[41] There is increasing evidence that the β-emitting ^{90}Y-octreotide will be effective in selected patients.

Medullary cancer cells are also relatively resistant to chemotherapy.[42] There is no single or combined chemotherapeutic protocol that provides statistically significant benefit. Protocols include adriamycin (doxorubicin) plus streptozocin, 5-fluorouracil plus dacarbazine, cyclophosphamide, vincristine, and dacarbazine, 5 fluorouracil/streptozocin and 5 fluorouracil/dacarbazine, or combined doxorubicin/streptozocin and 5 fluorouracil/dacarbazine.[43]

Medullary cancer cells exhibit somatostatin receptors and nonradioactive analogs of somatostatin. Octreotide has been prescribed by subcutaneous injection in a wide range of doses from 0.1 to 1.0 mg daily. Long-acting analogs have also been administered.[44] These agents stabilize or even lower calcitonin values but the growth of cancer is not slowed. The increasing knowledge of the molecular dysfunction in medullary cancer has led to experimental studies using inhibitors of tyrosine kinase such as Gleevec.[45] The data are conflicting.

The diarrhea can be treated by conventional medications including codeine. Capsaicin 0.25% applied locally helps cutaneous lichen amyloidosis. Cushing's syndrome caused by ectopic ACTH or its precursors can be helped by removal of the medullary cancer. In patients who have unresectable metastatic disease and severely symptomatic hyperadrenalism, it can be necessary to remove the adrenals.

There are rare reports of coexisting medullary and differentiated cancers; the latter are usually incidental and have been effectively treated by the thyroidectomy. When the differentiated cancer is large, invasive, or has metastasized, testing and treatment with radioiodine would follow the principles outlined in Chapter 5.

Follow-Up

Physical examination of the neck, measurement of calcitonin, CEA, and thyroid function, and ultrasound of the neck should be obtained at intervals of 6–12 months for several years. The hope is that calcitonin values remain low or undetectable. Minimally measurable values can be followed, but when the levels increase, the source of calcitonin production should be sought. Ultrasound of the entire neck is sensitive for identifying enlarged and abnormal-looking nodes and residual tissue in the thyroid bed. Ultrasound-guided FNA provides a tissue diagnosis. CT and MRI can be helpful, but after extensive surgery, postoperative scarring can be misinterpreted as cancer reducing the specificity of these tests. CT and MRI of the thorax and upper abdomen including the liver can identify disease in these sites. Miliary lesions in either organ exclude surgical treatment.

Scintigraphic Tests

Radionuclides of iodine are of no value in identifying local or distant metastases. MIBG labeled either by ^{131}I or ^{123}I is valuable for detecting pheochromocytoma but is less so for medullary cancer. ^{111}In-octreotide has been used for imaging.[46] Pentavalent dimercaptosuccinate labeled with technetium-

99m (^{99m}Tc) (^{99m}Tc-vDMSA) has been reported to have merit in detecting medullary cancer.[47] This is not available in the United States. Pentavalent-DMSA labeled with β emitters can be used to deliver local radiation to the cancer. ^{201}Tl and ^{99m}Tc-sestamibi and ^{99m}Tc-tetrafosmin are moderately successful.

^{18}Fluorodeoxyglucose (FDG)/PET has a sensitivity and specificity of approximately 80%.[48] Inflammatory diseases such as tuberculosis and sarcoidosis can give false positives.[49,50] Muscle uptake can occur in nervous patients or in those who talk or chew after injection of ^{18}FDG. In most cases, PET/CT allows the correct interpretation by providing an anatomic correlation for foci of uptake of ^{18}FDG.

Selective Venous Sampling

Measurement of calcitonin from venous sites in the neck can help define the site of residual or metastatic cancer. The technique requires a radiologist skilled in venous catheterization. The anatomy can be distorted by prior surgeries.

Prognosis

The prognosis is excellent when early identification and treatment of patients with a genetic predisposition to develop medullary cancer occur. In contrast, the outcome in a patient with distant metastases is very poor. Several other factors have a bearing on prognosis. Those factors that are statistically important as judged by univariate analysis are older age, the specific syndrome, stage of disease including the presence of metastases to lymph nodes and distant sites, and the completeness of the surgery. Women have a slightly better outcome. In the SEER report, the 5-year survivals were 83.8% in men and 92.8% in women and at 10 years the percentages were 74.3 and 89.6, respectively.[51] Patients with familial medullary cancer have the best prognosis followed by those with nonfamilial isolated medullary cancer, and those with MEN 2B have the worst outcome. A mutation in codons 883 and 918 predict a poorer outcome. Distant metastasis at the time of diagnosis is a bad feature. Cancers that are >4 cm also have a poorer outcome as do those with nodal metastases.

Summary

Medullary cancer is an uncommon thyroid cancer that arises from parafollicular C cells. The majority of medullary cancers are sporadic and they have the same mutations as familial syndromes but these are confined to the parafollicular cells. Sporadic cases should be diagnosed by FNA and treated by total thyroidectomy and central node dissection. About 25%–30% of medullary cancers are part of autosomal dominant familial syndromes such as familial medullary cancer, MEN 2A, and MEN 2B. Familial cases should be diagnosed early by genetic testing and the carriers treated by thyroidectomy at a young age. When the excised thyroid is normal or contains only C cell hyperplasia there should be no recurrence. Fifty percent of those with MEN syndromes will develop pheochromocytoma and 10%–25% of those with MEN 2A hyperparathyroidism; therefore, clinical follow-up and biochemical testing are necessary.

References

1. Donis-Keller H. The RET proto-oncogene and cancer. J Intern Med 1995;238(4): 319–325.
2. Bachelot A, Lombardo F, Baudin E, Bidart JM, Schlumberger M. Inheritable forms of medullary thyroid carcinoma. Biochimie 2002;84(1):61–66.
3. Caillou B, Rougier P, Schlumberger M, Talbot M, Parmentier C. Value of immunohistochemistry in the study of medullary cancer of the thyroid. Implications of the results for the concept of the APUD system and of apudomas. Bull Cancer 1984; 71(2):140–144.
4. Kebebew E, Ituarte PHG, Siperstein AE, Duh Q-Y, Clark OH. Medullary thyroid carcinoma. Clinical characteristics, treatment, prognostic factors, and a comparison of staging systems. Cancer 2000;88:1139–1148.
5. Ponder BA, Finer N, Coffey R, et al. Family screening in medullary thyroid carcinoma presenting without a family history. Q J Med 1988;67(252):299–308.
6. Ali SZ, Teichberg S, Attie JN, Susin M. Medullary thyroid carcinoma metastatic to breast masquerading as infiltrating lobular carcinoma. Ann Clin Lab Sci 1994; 24(5):441–447.
7. Jee MS, Chung YI, Lee MW, Choi JH, Moon KC, Koh JK. Cutaneous metastasis from medullary carcinoma of thyroid gland. Clin Exp Dermatol 2003;28(6):670–671.
8. Ordonez NG, Samaan NA. Medullary carcinoma of the thyroid metastatic to the skin: report of two cases. J Cutan Pathol 1987;14(4):251–254.
9. Puxeddu E, Fagin JA. Genetic markers in thyroid neoplasia. Endocrinol Metab Clin North Am 2001;30(2):493–513, x.
10. Graze K, Spiler IJ, Tashjian AH Jr, et al. Natural history of familial medullary thyroid carcinoma: effect of a program for early diagnosis. N Engl J Med 1978;299(18): 980–985.
11. Melvin K, Tashjian AH Jr. The syndrome of excessive thyrocalcitonin produced by medullary carcinoma of the thyroid. Proc Natl Acad Sci USA 1968;59:1216–1222.
12. Melvin KE, Tashjian AH Jr, Miller HH. Studies in familial (medullary) thyroid carcinoma. Recent Prog Horm Res 1972;28:399–470.

13. Elisei R, Bottici V, Luchetti F, et al. Impact of routine measurement of serum calcitonin on the diagnosis and outcome of medullary thyroid cancer: experience in 10,864 patients with nodular thyroid disorders. J Clin Endocrinol Metab 2004; 89(1):163–168.

14. Iacobone M, Niccoli-Sire P, Sebag F, De Micco C, Henry JF. Can sporadic medullary thyroid carcinoma be biochemically predicted? Prospective analysis of 66 operated patients with elevated serum calcitonin levels. World J Surg 2002;26(8):886–890.

15. Niccoli P, Conte-Devolx B, Lejeune PJ, et al. [Hypercalcitoninemia in conditions other than medullary cancers of the thyroid]. Ann Endocrinol (Paris) 1996;57(1): 15–21.

16. Schlumberger M, Pacini F. Medullary thyroid carcinoma. In: Schlumberger M, Pacini F, eds. Thyroid Tumors. Paris: Nucleon; 1999:267–299; 301–307.

17. Vierhapper H, Nowotny P, Bieglmayer Ch, Gessl A. Prevalence of hypergastrinemia in patients with hyper- and hypothyroidism: impact for calcitonin? Horm Res 2002;57(3–4):85–89.

18. Cooper DS, Doherty GM, Haugen BR, et al. Management guidelines for patients with thyroid nodules and differentiated thyroid cancer. Thyroid 2006;16(2):109–142.

19. Melvin KE, Tashjian AH Jr, Cassidy CE, Givens JR. Cushing's syndrome caused by ACTH- and calcitonin-secreting medullary carcinoma of the thyroid. Metabolism 1970;19(10):831–838.

20. Mure A, Gicquel C, Abdelmoumene N, et al. Cushing's syndrome in medullary thyroid carcinoma. J Endocrinol Invest 1995;18(3):180–185.

21. Smallridge RC, Bourne K, Pearson BW, Van Heerden JA, Carpenter PC, Young WF. Cushing's syndrome due to medullary thyroid carcinoma: diagnosis by proopiomelanocortin messenger ribonucleic acid in situ hybridization. J Clin Endocrinol Metab 2003;88(10):4565–4568.

22. Brandi M, Gagel RF, Angeli A, et al. Consensus: guidelines for diagnosis and therapy of MEN Type 1 and 2. J Clin Endocrinol Metab 2001;86:5658–5671.

23. NCCN. Practice Guidelines in Oncology. v. 1.2003. Thyroid Cancer: Medullary Cancer. CD available from National Comprehensive Cancer Network; 2004.

24. Yip L, Cote GJ, Shapiro SE, et al. Multiple endocrine neoplasia type 2: evaluation of the genotype-phenotype relationship. Arch Surg 2003;138(4):409–416; discussion 416.

25. Yen TW, Shapiro SE, Gagel RF, Sherman SI, Lee JE, Evans DB. Medullary thyroid carcinoma: results of a standardized surgical approach in a contemporary series of 80 consecutive patients. Surgery 2003;134(6):890–899; discussion 899–901.

26. Niccoli-Sire P, Murat A, Rohmer V, et al. When should thyroidectomy be performed in familial medullary thyroid carcinoma gene carriers with non-cysteine RET mutations? Surgery 2003;134(6):1029–1036; discussion 1036–1037.

27. Machens A, Niccoli-Sire P, Hoegel J, et al. Early malignant progression of hereditary medullary thyroid cancer. N Engl J Med 2003;349(16):1517–1525.

28. Pender S, Little DM, Burke P, Broe P. Treatment of medullary carcinoma of the thyroid by laryngo-pharyngo-oesophagectomy: a case report. Ir J Med Sci 1992; 161(7):450–451.

29. Saad MF, Guido JJ, Samaan NA. Radioactive iodine in the treatment of medullary carcinoma of the thyroid. J Clin Endocrinol Metab 1983;57(1):124–128.

30. Vitale G, Caraglia M, Ciccarelli A, Lupoli G, Abbruzzese A, Tagliaferri P. Current approaches and perspectives in the therapy of medullary thyroid carcinoma. Cancer 2001;91(9):1797–1808.

31. Bellantone R, Boscherini M, Lombardi CP, Alesina PF. Medullary thyroid carcinoma: surgical management of primary tumor and locoregional recurrence. Rays 2000;25(2):267–271.

32. Pollinger B, Duhmke E. External radiotherapy of thyroid cancer. Onkologie 2001; 24(2):134–138.

33. Simpson WJ, Palmer JA, Rosen IB, Mustard RA. Management of medullary carcinoma of the thyroid. Am J Surg 1982;144(4):420–422.

34. Tubiana M, Haddad E, Schlumberger M, Hill C, Rougier P, Sarrazin D. External radiotherapy in thyroid cancers. Cancer 1985;55(suppl 9):2062–2071.

35. Sarrazin D, Fontaine F, Rougier P, et al. [Role of radiotherapy in the treatment of medullary cancer of the thyroid]. Bull Cancer 1984;71(3):200–208.

36. Hoefnagel CA, Delprat CC, Valdes Olmos RA. Role of [131]metaiodobenzylguanidine therapy in medullary thyroid carcinoma. J Nucl Biol Med 1991;35(4):334–336.

37. Castellani MR, Alessi A, Savelli G, Bombardieri E. The role of radionuclide therapy in medullary thyroid cancer. Tumori 2003;89(5):560–562.

38. Wiseman GA, Kvols LK. Therapy of neuroendocrine tumors with radiolabeled MIBG and somatostatin analogues. Semin Nucl Med 1995;25(3):272–278.

39. Shapiro B. Ten years of experience with MIBG applications and the potential of new radiolabeled peptides: a personal overview and concluding remarks. Q J Nucl Med 1995;39(4 suppl 1):150–155.

40. Juweid ME, Hajjar G, Stein R, et al. Initial experience with high-dose radioimmunotherapy of metastatic medullary thyroid cancer using 131I-MN-14 F(ab)2 anti-carcinoembryonic antigen MAb and AHSCR. J Nucl Med 2000;41(1):93–103.

41. Forssell-Aronsson EB, Nilsson O, Bejegard SA, et al. 111In-DTPA-D-Phe1-octreotide binding and somatostatin receptor subtypes in thyroid tumors. J Nucl Med 2000; 41(4):636–642.

42. Yang KP, Liang YF, Samaan NA. Intrinsic drug resistance in a human medullary thyroid carcinoma cell line: association with overexpression of mdr1 gene and low proliferation fraction. Anticancer Res 1991;11(3):1065–1068.

43. Nocera M, Baudin E, Pellegriti G, Cailleux AF, Mechelany-Corone C, Schlumberger M. Treatment of advanced medullary thyroid cancer with an alternating combination of doxorubicin-streptozocin and 5 FU-dacarbazine. Groupe d'Etude des Tumeurs a Calcitonine (GETC). Br J Cancer 2000;83(6):715–718.

44. Ahlman H, Tisell LE. The use of a long-acting somatostatin analogue in the treatment of advanced endocrine malignancies with gastrointestinal symptoms. Scand J Gastroenterol 1987;22(8):938–942.

45. Lanzi C, Cassinelli G, Cuccuru G, Zanchi C, Laccabue D, Zunino F. RET/PTC oncoproteins: molecular targets of new drugs. Tumori 2003;89(5):520–522.

46. Zhang J, Dai W, Lian X, et al. [Detection of remnants after removal of medullary thyroid carcinoma]. Zhonghua Wai Ke Za Zhi 2000;38(1):19–21.

47. Adams BK, Fataar A, Byrne MJ, Levitt NS, Matley PJ. Pentavalent technetium-99m (V)-DMSA uptake in a pheochromocytoma in a patient with Sipple's syndrome. J Nucl Med 1990;31(1):106–108.

48. Bockisch A, Brandt-Mainz K, Gorges R, Muller S, Stattaus J, Antoch G. Diagnosis in medullary thyroid cancer with [18F]FDG-PET and improvement using a combined PET/CT scanner. Acta Med Austriaca 2003;30(1):22–25.

49. Cook G, Maisey MN, Fogelman I. Normal variants, artefacts and interpretative pitfalls in PET with 18-fluoro-2-deoxyglucose and carbon-11 methionine. Eur J Nucl Med 1999;26:1363–1378.

50. Shreve PD, Anzai Y, Wahl RL. Pitfalls in oncologic diagnosis with FDG PET imaging: physiologic and benign variants. Radiographics 1999;19(1):61–77; quiz 150–151.

51. Bhattacharyya N. A population-based analysis of survival factors in differentiated and medullary thyroid carcinoma. Otolaryngol Clin North Am 2003;128:115–125.

11. Primary Lymphoma of the Thyroid

Primary lymphoma of the thyroid is uncommon. Physicians caring for patients with thyroid diseases will occasionally encounter one with primary lymphoma in the thyroid. In almost all of these patients, the pathology demonstrates non-Hodgkin's lymphoma. Most patients with primary lymphoma of the thyroid are older women, many of whom have previously been diagnosed with Hashimoto's thyroiditis. Rapid enlargement of the thyroid and local pressure effects are common.

Pathology

Lymphoma of the thyroid is usually non-Hodgkin's B cell lymphoma.[1–5] A proportion of these cancers are derived from mucosal-associated lymphocytes and known by the abbreviation MALT.[6] Approximately 1 of 200 patients with Hashimoto's thyroiditis develop lymphoma. This means the association is uncommon; however, it is 67 times the expected incidence of lymphoma of the thyroid in the population.

Clinical Features

Seventy-five percent of patients are women and the average age is 60–70 years. There is rapid growth of the thyroid, or enlargement of a nodule within the thyroid or a previously stable goiter of Hashimoto's thyroiditis. Pressure effects on the aerodigestive tract occur, commonly causing dyspnea, stridor, and dysphagia. The voice can become hoarse from entrapment of the recurrent laryngeal nerve. Pain is uncommon. Symptoms of weight loss, fever, and weakness occur in about 10% of patients. The gland is hard and irregular on palpation and there can be fixation to surrounding soft tissues of the neck. Thyroid function is usually normal, but can be low because of Hashimoto's thyroiditis. Thyrotoxicosis results from release of stored thyroid hormones by invasive cancer but this is rare.

Diagnosis

Fine needle aspiration (FNA) and interpretation of the cytology and use of flow cytometry and immunophenotyping of the lymphocytes establish the diagnosis.[7] Differentiation of a low-grade lymphoma from Hashimoto's thyroiditis is not possible by cytomorphology alone but is usually possible with immunophenotyping. With increasingly improving molecular techniques, open biopsy should be used less frequently.[7] Differential diagnoses include goitrous Hashimoto's thyroiditis and anaplastic thyroid cancer.[8]

Workup of Patient

Scintigraphy and ultrasound do not help establish the correct diagnosis. However, ultrasound can be helpful in determining the optimal site for FNA sampling and the key is to obtain a tissue diagnosis. Staging of the lymphoma should be under the direction of an expert in the management of lymphoma. It is stressed that the clinical features of a rapidly growing nodule or goiter in an older woman should prompt FNA to establish a tissue diagnosis. Treatment should never be based on the imaging findings alone. Positron emission tomography (PET)/computed tomography is useful for staging but is less helpful for diagnosis of the primary cancer because there is often fluorodeoxy-glucose (FDG) uptake in uncomplicated Hashimoto's thyroiditis (Figure 11.1).[9–11]

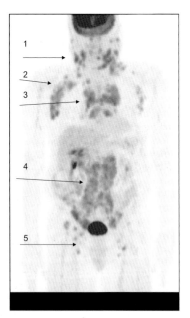
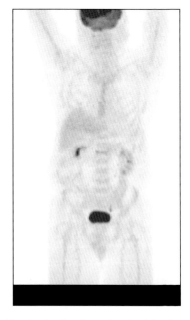

Figure 11.1. A [18]FDG PET scan in a patient with extensive lymphoma (not involving the thyroid). There is uptake of FDG in almost all lymph nodes. **B** The same patient after chemotherapy demonstrating remarkable resolution of the lymphoma.

Management

Treatment and follow-up are usually directed by a medical oncologist, or in some cases, a radiation oncologist. The chemotherapeutic regimes and indications for external radiation therapy are outside the scope of this text. After treatment with combination chemotherapy, 5- and 10-year survivals are 75%–80% and 50%–60%, respectively.[12,13]

Summary and Key Facts

Primary lymphoma of the thyroid is rare and it usually occurs in an older woman who has had Hashimoto's thyroiditis. Once the diagnosis is established by FNA, the patient should be referred to an oncology center specializing in the care of lymphoma.

References

1. Sirota DK, Segal RL. Primary lymphomas of the thyroid gland. JAMA 1979; 242(16):1743–1746.
2. Soltes SF. Primary malignant lymphoma of the thyroid. Ear Nose Throat J 1981; 60(3):131–135.
3. Matsuzuka F, Miyauchi A, Katayama S, et al. Clinical aspects of primary thyroid lymphoma: diagnosis and treatment based on our experience of 119 cases. Thyroid 1993;3(2):93–99.
4. Schwarze EW, Papadimitriou C. Malignant lymphomas of the thyroid gland (author's transl). Verh Dtsch Ges Pathol 1977;61:328–335.
5. Devine RM, Edis AJ, Banks PM. Primary lymphoma of the thyroid: a review of the Mayo Clinic experience through 1978. World J Surg 1981;5(1):33–38.
6. Fonseca E, Sambade C. Primary lymphomas of the thyroid gland: a review with emphasis on diagnostic features. Arch Anat Cytol Pathol 1998;46(1–2):94–99.
7. Detweiler RE, Katz RL, Alapat C, el-Naggar A, Ordonez N. Malignant lymphoma of the thyroid: a report of two cases diagnosed by fine-needle aspiration. Diagn Cytopathol 1991;7(2):163–171.
8. Ishikawa H, Tamaki Y, Takahashi M, et al. Comparison of primary thyroid lymphoma with anaplastic thyroid carcinoma on computed tomographic imaging. Radiat Med 2002;20(1):9–15.
9. Chander S, Zingas AP, Bloom DA, Zak IT, Joyrich RN, Getzen TM. Positron emission tomography in primary thyroid lymphoma. Clin Nucl Med 2004;29(9):572–573.
10. Yasuda S, Ide M, Takagi S, Shohtsu A. [Cancer screening with whole-body FDG PET]. Kaku Igaku 1996;33(10):1065–1071.

11. Yasuda S, Shohtsu A, Ide M, et al. Chronic thyroiditis: diffuse uptake of FDG at PET. Radiology 1998;207:775–778.

12. Thieblemont C, Mayer A, Dumontet C, et al. Primary thyroid lymphoma is a heterogeneous disease. J Clin Endocrinol Metab 2002;87(1):105–111.

13. Sippel RS, Gauger PG, Angelos P, Thompson NW, Mack E, Chen H. Palliative thyroidectomy for malignant lymphoma of the thyroid. Ann Surg Oncol 2002; 9(9):907–911.

12. Metastases to the Thyroid

Based on its size, the thyroid has the second highest arterial blood flow. Therefore, it can be the site of blood-borne metastases. Systemic metastases are usually found in the lungs, liver, brain, and bone marrow, and certain cancers have a natural propensity to metastasize to specific sites such as prostate cancer to the skeleton and bowel cancer to the liver. Common cancers seldom metastasize to the thyroid. When a nonthyroidal cancer is diagnosed in the thyroid, the key is how should the patient be managed?

Incidence of Metastases to the Thyroid at Autopsy

Two reports indicate that at autopsy between 5.2% and 8.6% of patients with nonthyroidal cancer have thyroidal metastases.[1,2] There is a wide range from 1.25% in unselected patients to 24.2% in selected patients with known metastatic cancer. The range is likely attributable to the population under consideration and the extent to which the pathologist searches.

Clinical Importance of Metastases

When a patient who has widespread metastases of nonthyroidal cancer is found to have a new thyroid mass, the implication is that it is also a metastasis. However, there is no benefit from proving that the thyroid nodule is a metastasis because neither treatment nor outcome is changed. In contrast, when a patient with a known cancer but no evidence of metastases develops a thyroid nodule, this might be a solitary metastasis.[3] Metastasis to the thyroid can occur many years after treatment of the primary lesion. For example, 12 of 43 patients developed the thyroid metastasis more than 10 years after the original diagnosis of cancer.[4] Two separate case reports are of metastasis 14 and 19 years after nephrectomy for renal cancer.[5,6] A third clinical situation is a fine needle aspiration (FNA) result that is consistent with metastasis but the patient has no history of cancer and no other metastases. This presentation is "carcinoma (usually adenocarcinoma) of unknown origin." In two reports of metastases to the thyroid, 16 of 21 and 5 of 15 patients had no prior diagnosis of cancer.[7,8]

The metastasis to the thyroid can grow rapidly and cause compression of the aerodigestive tract. It might invade and destroy normal thyroid and produce biochemical and or clinical thyrotoxicosis.[9] This is called carcinomatous pseudothyroiditis and is difficult to differentiate from subacute thyroiditis. FNA is recommended when a patient with cancer presents with a painful thyroid mass and thyrotoxicosis. In addition, in an elderly patient with atypical clinical features of subacute thyroiditis, FNA is indicated.

Diagnosis of Metastasis to the Thyroid

Most of the patients are older than 50 years of age and the genders are about equal, and a new thyroid nodule is identified by clinical examination or imaging. A tissue diagnosis by FNA should be obtained quickly. Most benign and malignant nodules are nonfunctioning on scintiscan, therefore this is not advised.[10,11] Ultrasound is not specific because almost all metastases appear as ill-defined, heterogeneous, hypoechoic masses. Ultrasound is not recommended for diagnosis but can help in conducting the FNA. When the FNA result indicates a nonthyroidal carcinoma, a review of prior surgeries and pathologies can help clarify the diagnosis.

The vast majority of metastases to the thyroid are from five primary cancers: kidney, lung, breast, gastrointestinal tract, and melanoma, as shown in Table 12.1. The number of kidney lesions is disproportionate to the incidence of that cancer. The presence of suspected metastatic renal cancer to the thyroid raises a dilemma because clear cell cancer of the kidney cannot always be easily differentiated from clear cell follicular cancer. On FNA and histologic specimens, staining for organ-specific antigens should be part of the diagnostic process.

Uncommon cancers can metastasize to the thyroid but this is extremely rare and these are usually reported as single case reports. They include chromophobe renal cell cancer, choriocarcinoma, uterine leiomyosarcoma, pancreatic cancer, squamous cell cancer of the mouth, adrenal cancer, bronchioalveolar cancer, colon cancer, rectal carcinoid, sarcoma, Kaposi's sarcoma, liposarcoma, and malignant fibrous histiocytoma, and are referenced in McDougall[12] and Haugen et al.[13] Metastases seem to be more frequent in patients with underlying thyroid disorders such as nodular thyroids.[14] There are even reports of renal cancer and a colon cancer that metastasized to Hürthle cell cancers.

Table 12.1. Percentage (and ranges) of nonthyroidal metastases from five key primary cancers (for details, see reference 12)

	Kidney (%)	Breast (%)	Lung (%)	Gastrointestinal tract (%)	Melanoma (%)
12 reports	32 (12–56)	30 (7–67)	26 (7–50)	14 (7–24)	10 (3–25)

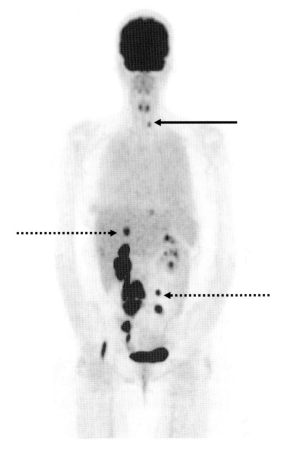

Figure 12.1. PET scan using ^{18}fluorodeoxyglucose in a patient with bowel cancer. Focal uptake in thyroid (solid arrow) is a metastasis from that cancer. The patient also has metastases to abdominal lymph nodes and the liver (one of each shown by dotted arrow).

Treatment of a Metastasis to the Thyroid

Treatment depends on the extent of the metastatic disease. There is no reason to investigate a new thyroid nodule in a dying patient. However, a new thyroid nodule in a healthy patient with a known primary cancer should be investigated using FNA to determine the pathology. FNA might demonstrate a benign thyroid nodule, a primary thyroid cancer, or a metastasis. In the case of metastasis, long-term survival is possible after removal of the thyroidal lesion, especially in renal cancer.[4,15,16] Isolated metastasis from melanoma can also be treated surgically.[16] It is important to "stage" the cancer to ensure there are no other unsuspected lesions. Computed tomography (CT) of the chest, abdomen, and pelvis are obtained plus positron emission tomography (PET)/CT, which has excellent sensitivity for most common cancers (Figure 12.1).[17]

When the FNA of a thyroid nodule is reported to be a metastatic cancer but the patient is not known to have cancer, it is necessary to identify the primary site. The cytologic findings might help direct the appropriate workup. Should this not be helpful, clinical examination of the skin and imaging of the kidneys, lung, and breast would be advised along with CT of chest and abdomen and mammography. PET/CT is valuable in patients with carcinoma of unknown origin.[18] When the metastasis to the thyroid is the only lesion, surgical removal of the primary cancer and thyroid including the metastasis can prolong survival and even be curative.[19] Before major surgery is undertaken, it should be clear that there is significant life expectancy of good quality. The site, size, and pathology of the primary cancer, the extent of metastases, the patient's age, and state of general health all have to be considered. When extensive metastases are present, chemotherapy appropriate for the primary cancer is administered. External radiation therapy is delivered to painful or expanding lesions. When the primary cancer is not identified, patients are treated by protocols for the most likely "adenocarcinoma of unknown origin."

Prognosis

The prognosis varies greatly depending on the patient's clinical presentation. Survival longer than a few months is not expected when there are multiple metastases. An isolated metastasis that can be surgically excised can result in longer survival. Of 37 patients, the average survival was 34 months in those who had thyroidectomy versus 25 months in those who did not.[4] Ten patients with renal cell metastases to the thyroid who underwent "metastectomy" survived an average of 39 months. In a second report, the average survival in seven patients after thyroidectomy was 38 months.[20]

Summary and Key Points

The reported incidence of metastases to the thyroid varies widely, the highest in patients dying with disseminated disease whose thyroids are examined carefully at postmortem. Kidney, breast, lung, gastrointestinal cancers, and melanoma have a propensity to metastasize to the thyroid. A thyroidal metastasis is rarely the first evidence of a nonthyroidal cancer. FNA is the best first investigation. The extent of disease should be determined, and when the thyroidal metastasis is the only distant lesion, removal of the primary and the thyroid can result in long-term survival. This should not be attempted when there is evidence of extensive spread of cancer.

References

1. Willis R. Metastatic tumors in the thyroid. Am J Pathol 1931;7:187–208.
2. Shimaoka K, Sokal J, Pickren J. Metastatic neoplasms in the thyroid gland. Cancer 1962;15:557–565.
3. McCabe D, Farrar WB, Petkov TM, Finkelmeier W, O'Dwyer P, James A. Clinical and pathologic correlations in disease metastatic to the thyroid gland. Am J Surg 1985;150:519–523.
4. Nakhjavani MK, Gharib H, Goellner JR, van Heerden JA. Metastasis to the thyroid gland. A report of 43 cases. Cancer 1997;79(3):574–578.
5. Kihara M, Yokomise H, Yamauchi A. Metastasis of renal cell carcinoma to the thyroid gland 19 years after nephrectomy: a case report. Auris Nasus Larynx 2004; 31(1):95–100.
6. Pereira Arias JG, Acinas Garcia O, Escobal Tamayo V, et al. [Late metastasis in thyroid gland after nephrectomy for renal clear cell carcinoma]. Actas Urol Esp 1995;19(6):468–472.
7. Michelow PM, Leiman G. Metastases to the thyroid gland: diagnosis by aspiration cytology. Diagn Cytopathol 1995;13(3):209–213.
8. Wood K, Vini L, Harmer C. Metastases to the thyroid gland: the Royal Marsden experience. Eur J Surg Oncol 2004;30(6):583–588.
9. De Ridder M, Sermeus AB, Urbain D, Storme GA. Metastases to the thyroid gland: a report of six cases. Eur J Intern Med 2003;14(6):377–379.
10. Ahuja AT, King W, Metreweli C. Role of ultrasonography in thyroid metastases. Clin Radiol 1994;49(9):627–629.
11. Chung S, Kim E-K, Kim JH, et al. Sonographic findings of metastatic disease to the thyroid. Yonsei Med J 2001;42:411–417.
12. McDougall I. Management of Thyroid Cancer and Related Nodular Diseases. London: Springer-Verlag; 2006:Chapter 12.
13. Haugen B, Nawaz S, Cohn A, et al. Secondary malignancy of the thyroid gland: a case report and review of the literature. Thyroid 1994;4:297–300.
14. Ro JY, Guerrieri C, el-Naggar AK, Ordonez NG, Sorge JG, Ayala AG. Carcinomas metastatic to follicular adenomas of the thyroid gland. Report of two cases. Arch Pathol Lab Med 1994;118(5):551–556.
15. Heffess CS, Wenig BM, Thompson LD. Metastatic renal cell carcinoma to the thyroid gland: a clinicopathologic study of 36 cases. Cancer 2002;95(9):1869–1878.
16. Ericsson M, Biorklund A, Cederquist E, Ingemansson S, Akerman M. Surgical treatment of metastatic disease in the thyroid gland. J Surg Oncol 1981;17(1):15–23.
17. Gambhir S, Czernin J, Schwimmer J, Silverman DHS, Coleman RE, Phelps ME. A tabulated summary of the FDG PET literature. J Nucl Med 2001;42:1S–93S.

18. Goerres G. PET and PET/CT of tumors with an unknown primary. In: van Schulthess GK, ed. Clinical Molecular Anatomic Imaging. Philadelphia: Lippincott Williams & Wilkins; 2003:284–290.

19. May M, Marusch F, Kaufmann O, et al. [Solitary renal cell carcinoma metastasis to the thyroid gland—a paradigm of metastasectomy?]. Chirurg 2003;74(8):768–774.

20. Benoit L, Favoulet P, Arnould L, et al. [Metastatic renal cell carcinoma of the thyroid gland: about seven cases and review of the literature]. Ann Chir 2004;129(4): 218–223.

Index

Printed in Singapore